INTRO

If you are like me, you have a family, household and business to run, and squeezing in a solid 30 minute workout seems daunting most days. This book is to encourage you to get workouts in throughout your day, whenever you can squeeze them in.

I am not a fitness instructor or licensed anything. I'm just a Graphic Designer that wanted to make a pretty book to encourage others to incorporate fun exercises into their day like I do. So consult your doctor prior to starting an exercise regime, especially if you have underlining medical conditions.

Alicia

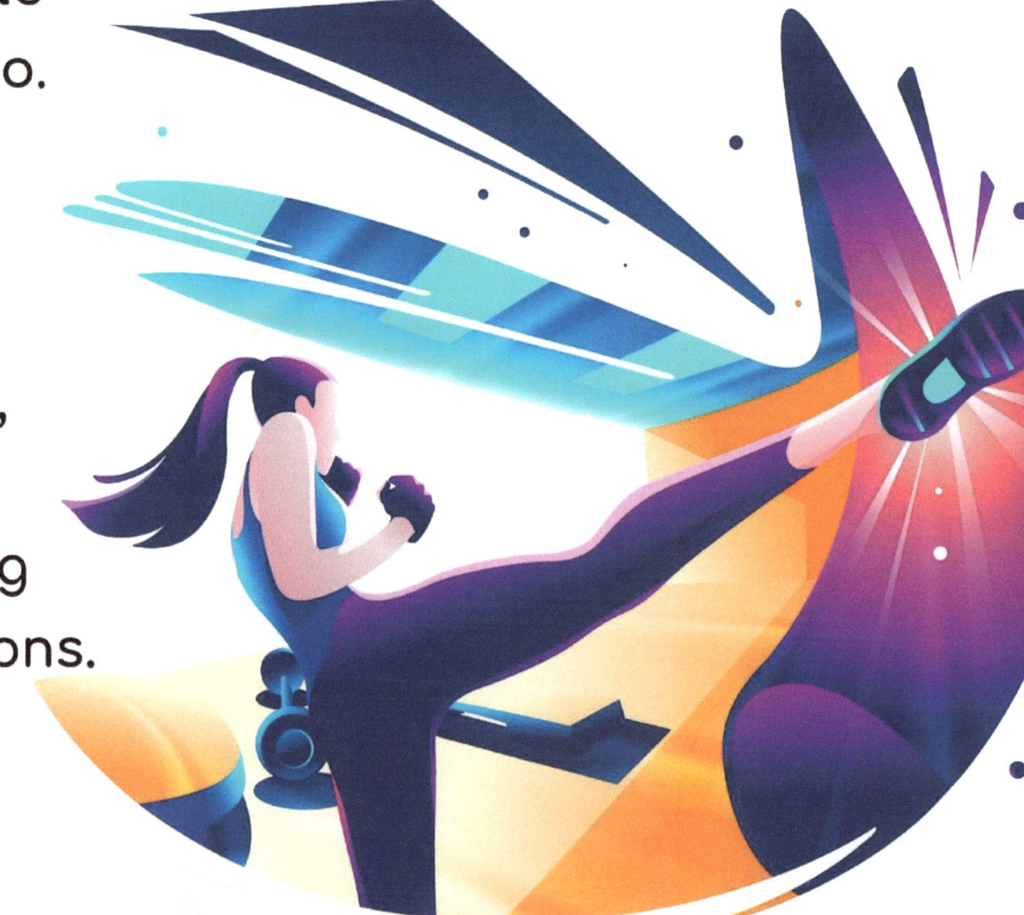

HOW TO USE THE BOOK

(Do online searches if you need more information on proper forms for specific exercises.)

1. **No equipment needed**, but if you have, that's great. It will boost your workouts.

2. **Flip through the book at your own leisure** and put your entire effort into each workout. Lazy movements won't get results.

3. **If something doesn't feel right - stop**. No one knows your body like you do.

4. **Always take care of your** knees, core and lower back during exercises. Hold your core (abs) tight in workouts, to protect your spine.

Are you advanced and want to do the entire book in one workout?
IT WILL TAKE YOU 50–60 MINS

NOW, LET'S GO MAKE OUR FAT CRY!

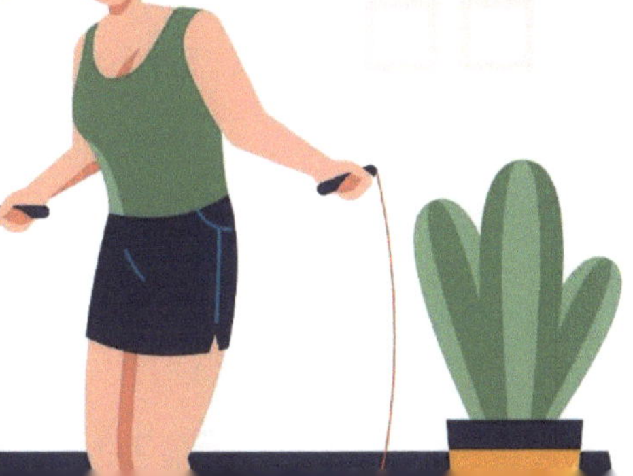

TABLE OF CONTENTS

(All workouts are colour-coded throughout the book, for ease of use.)

WORKOUT

1

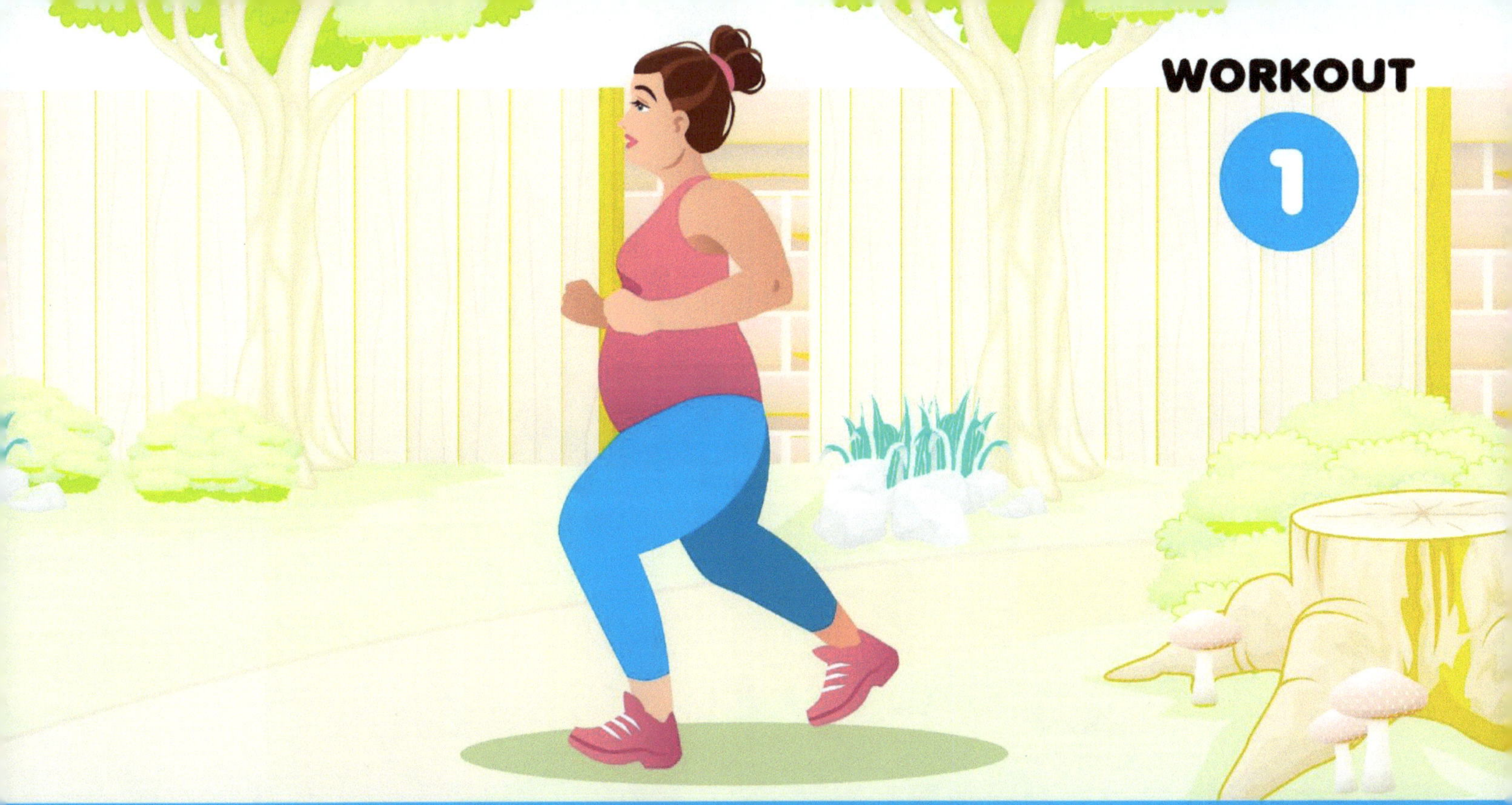

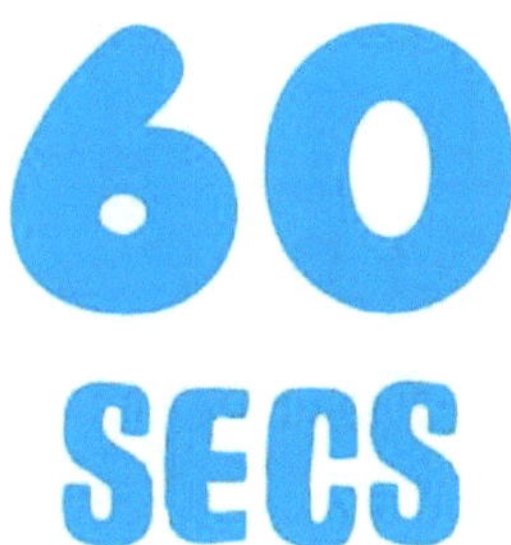

RUN ON THE SPOT

HOW LONG?

60

SECS

HOW TO DO IT

Run, jog, march or
air jump rope on the spot.

Run like the wind, even though
you might just be the breeze.

READY FOR THE NEXT ONE? ➡

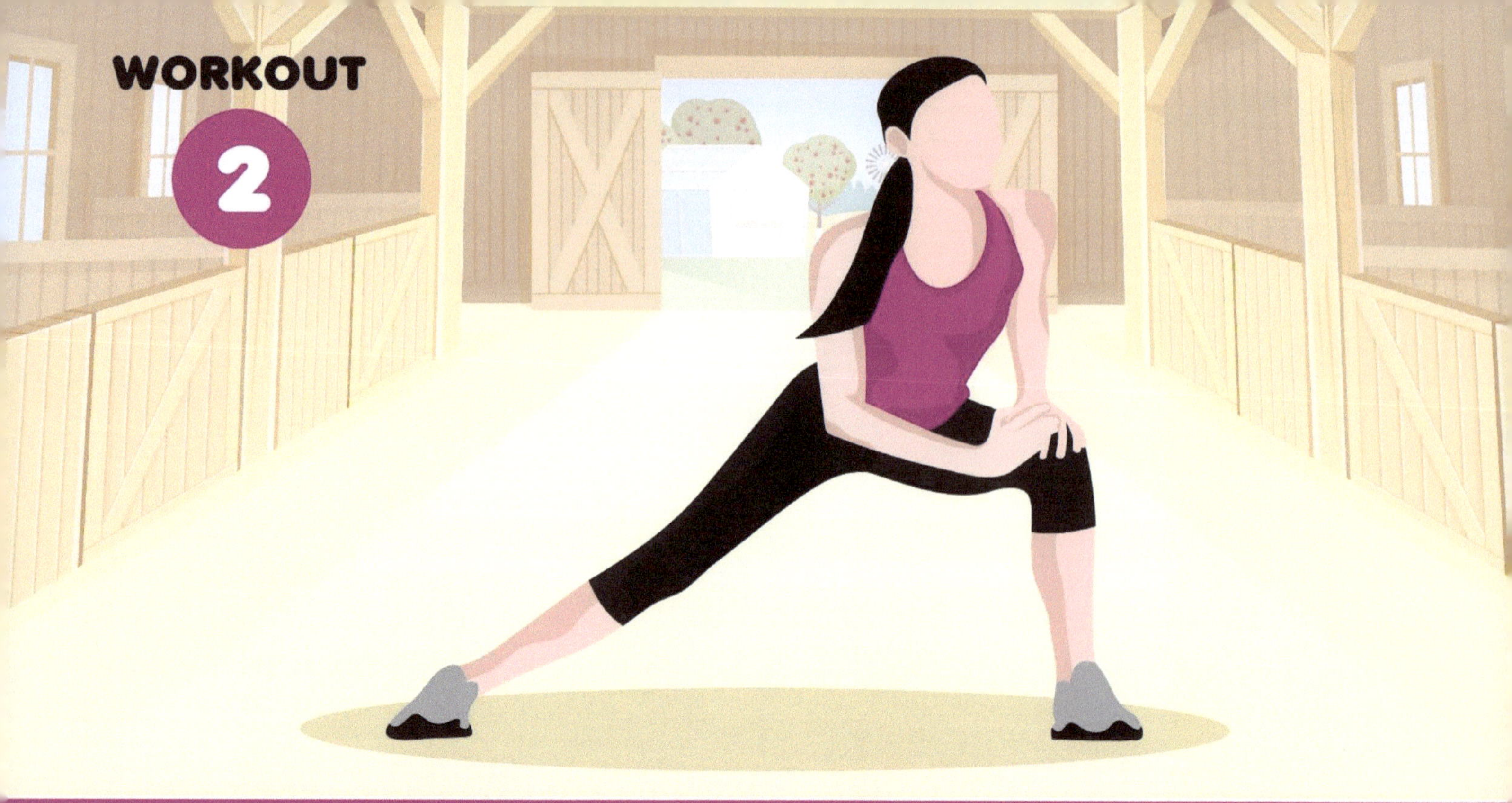

SIDE LUNGE STRETCH

HOW MANY?

14

TOTAL

HOW TO DO IT

Standing, lunge to the side and lean lightly on your knee. After 2 seconds, switch sides.

This is a dynamic stretch, so continuous movement from side-to-side is key here.

READY FOR THE NEXT ONE? 

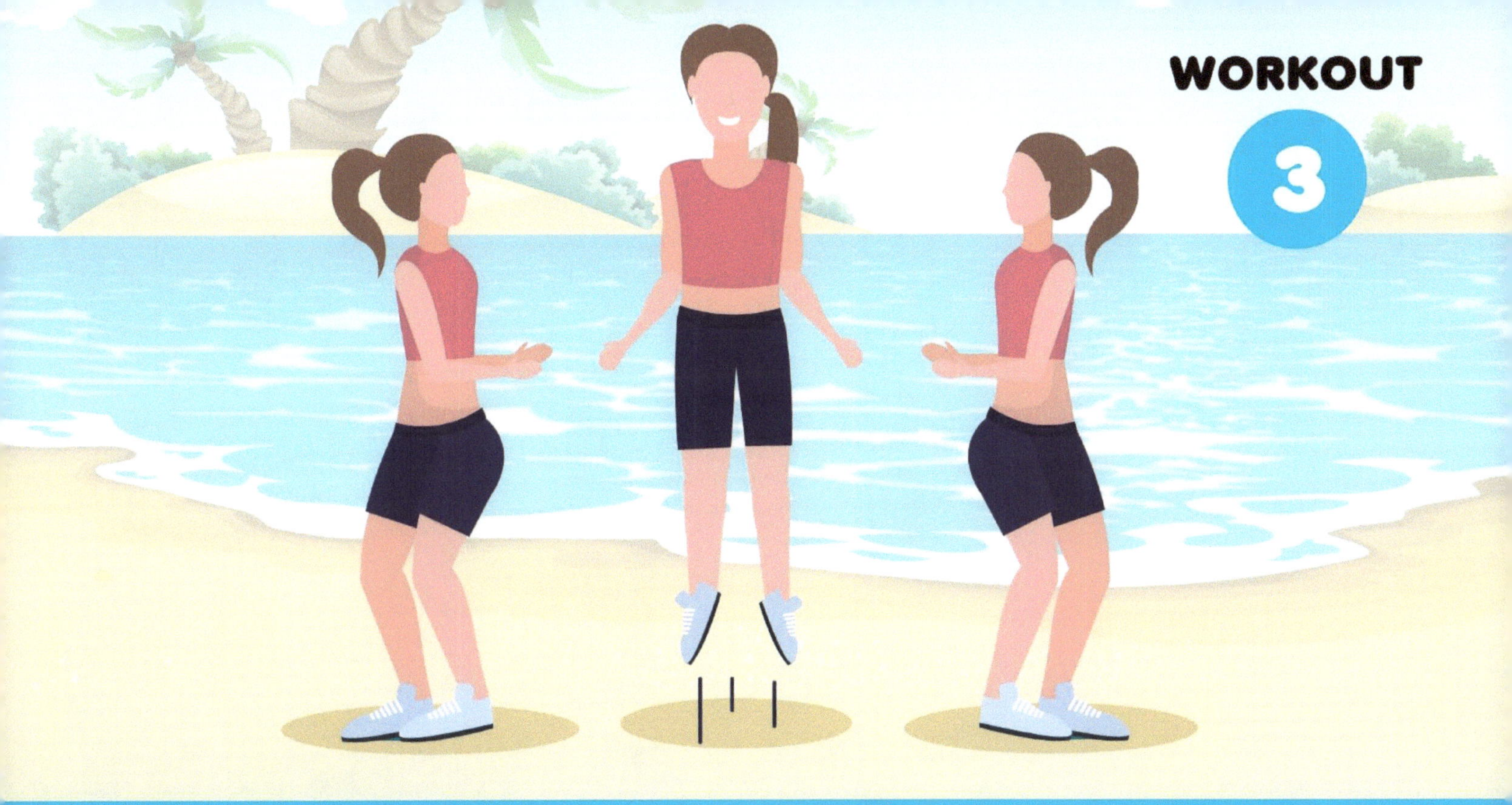

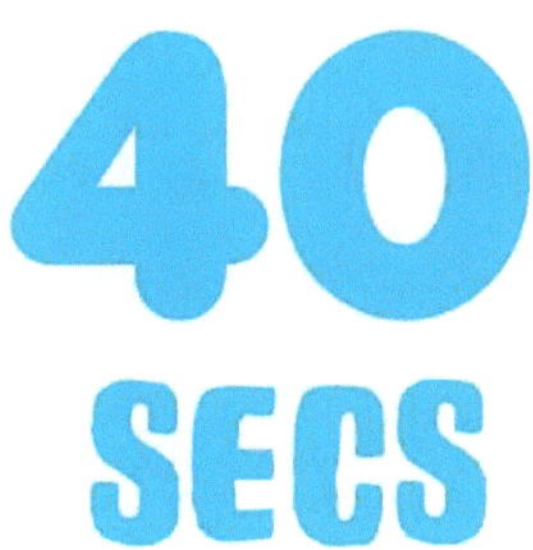

SKIERS

HOW LONG?

40 SECS

HOW TO DO IT

4 jumps continuously. Front, right, front, left. The upper body position should twist in the opposite direction on the side jumps.

You can do this on ground or skiing down a 4000 foot mountain slope. Your choice.

READY FOR THE NEXT ONE? 

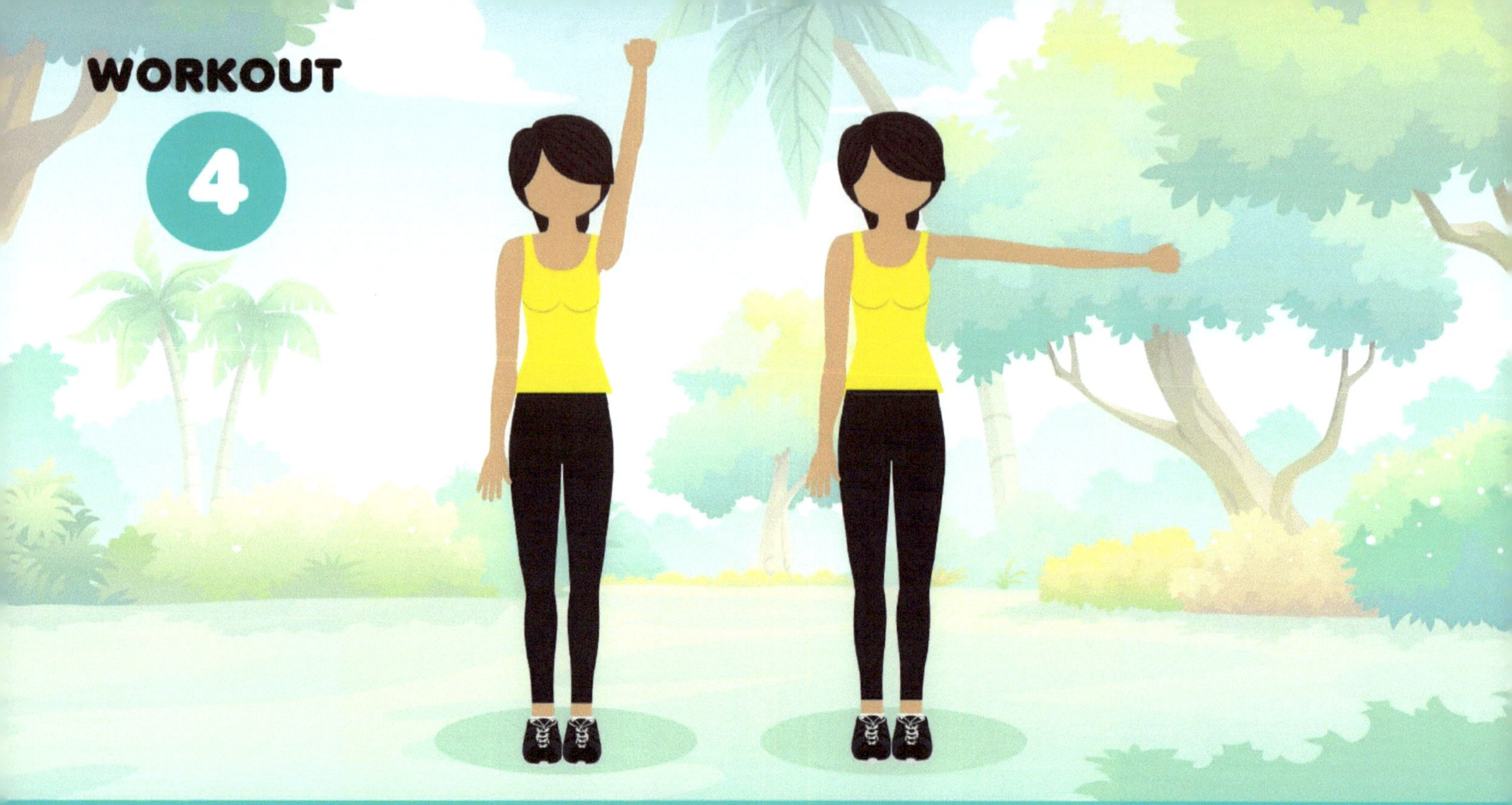

SKY AND SIDE PUNCH

HOW MANY?

15

EACH SIDE

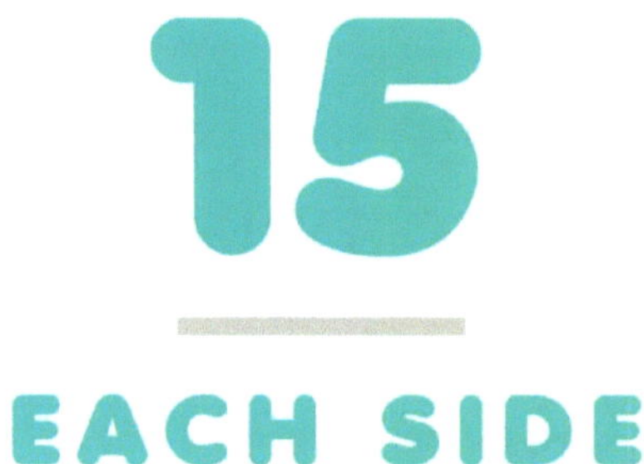

HOW TO DO IT

Punch up to the sky and then punch out to the side with the same arm.

Cardio for your arm fat.

READY FOR THE NEXT ONE? 

WORKOUT

5

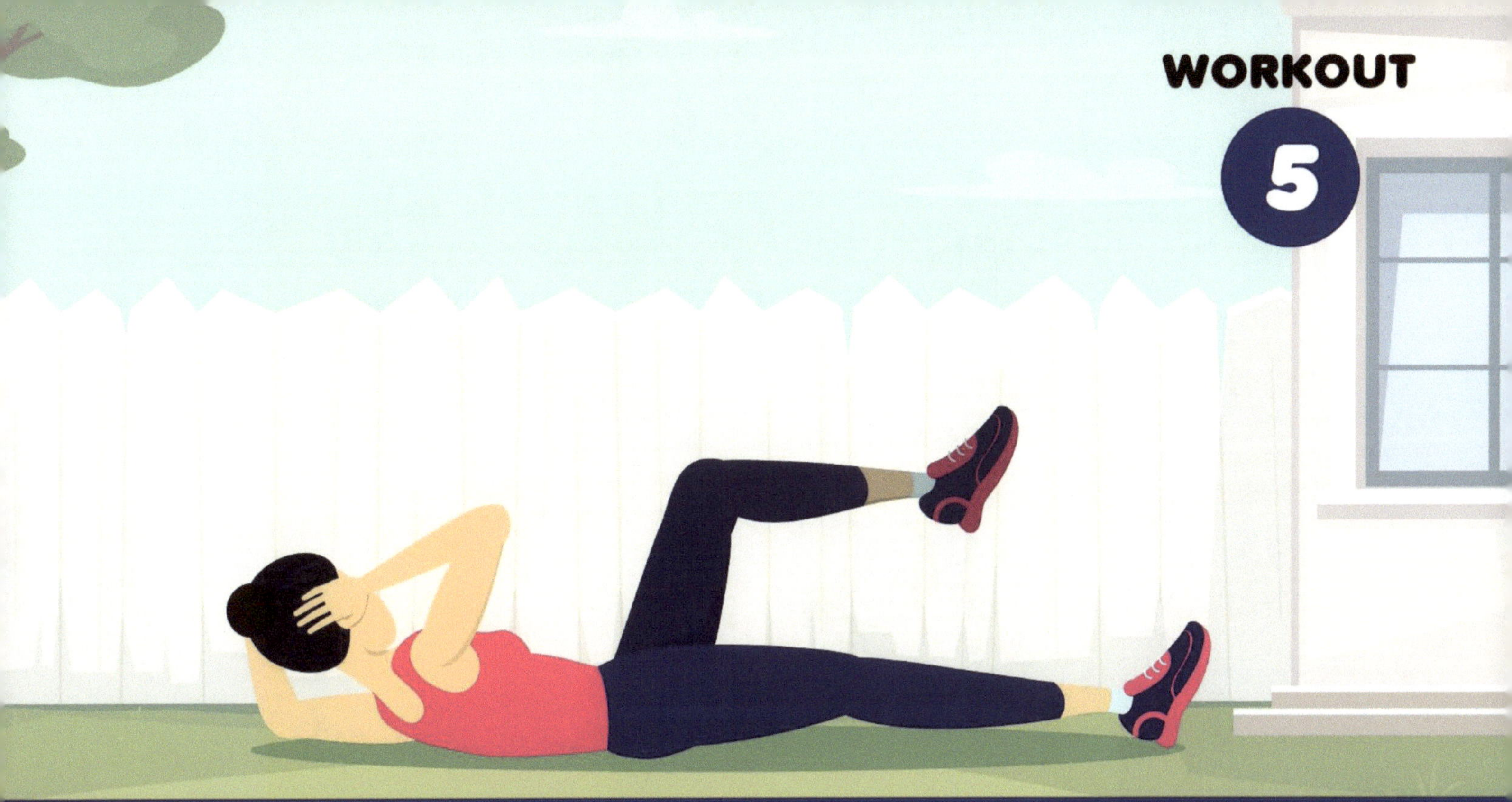

BICYCLE CRUNCHES

HOW MANY?

20

TOTAL

HOW TO DO IT

Starting flat on your back, hands behind head, lift your head as opposite elbow reaches opposite knee. Alternate back and forth quickly.

The workout that will create abs of steel.

READY FOR THE NEXT ONE? →

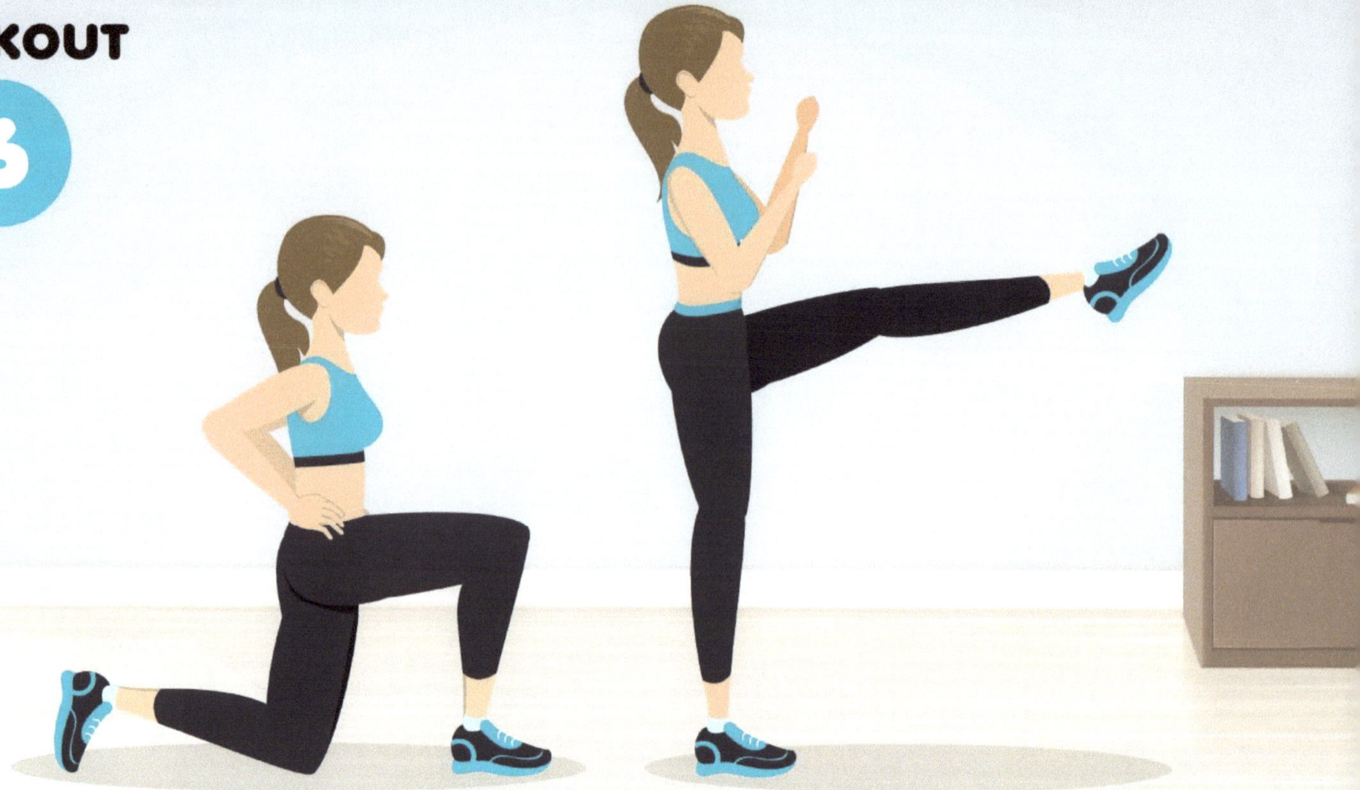

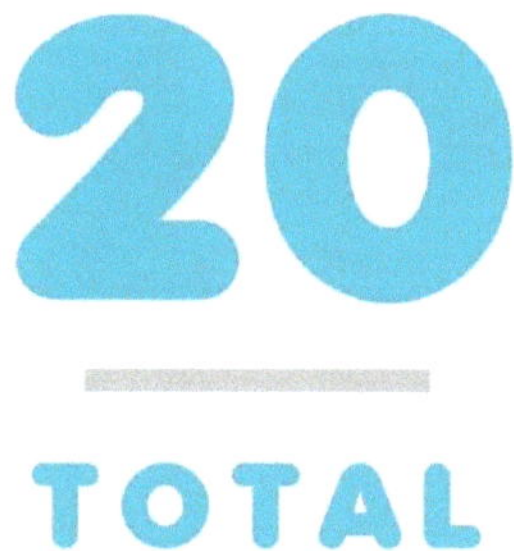

REVERSE LUNGE KICKS

HOW MANY?

20

TOTAL

HOW TO DO IT

Standing, step back and drop your knee towards the ground. Stand, then front kick that same leg. Alternate.

Exercise is like a relationship, you can't cheat and expect it to work.

READY FOR THE NEXT ONE? 

WORKOUT

7

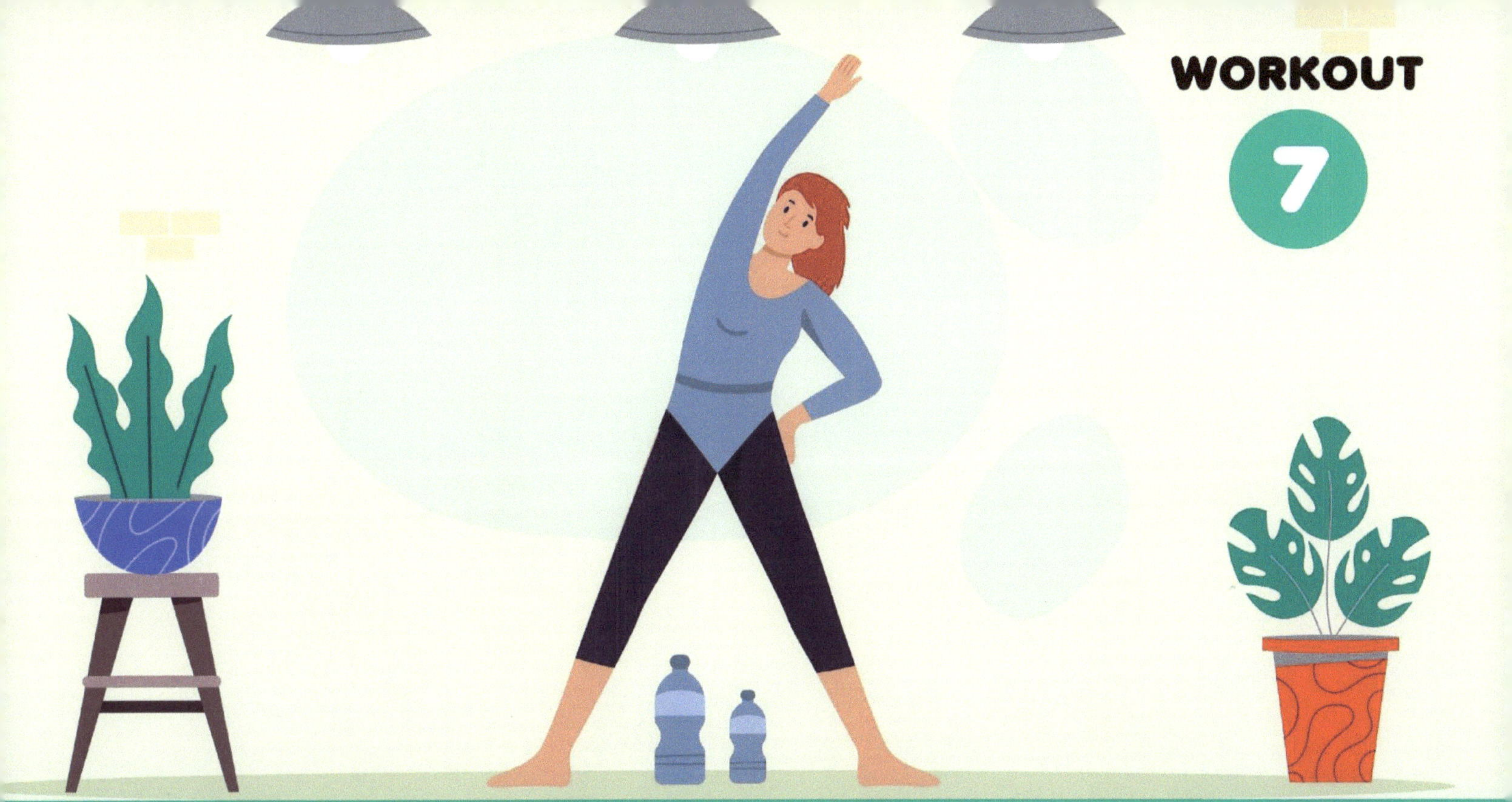

ARM REACHES

HOW MANY?

6

TOTAL

HOW TO DO IT

With feet slightly apart, lean to the side, stretching a straight arm to the sky. Hold for 5 seconds. Alternate.

Stretch like you're checking if your deodorant is still working.

READY FOR THE NEXT ONE?

WORKOUT

8

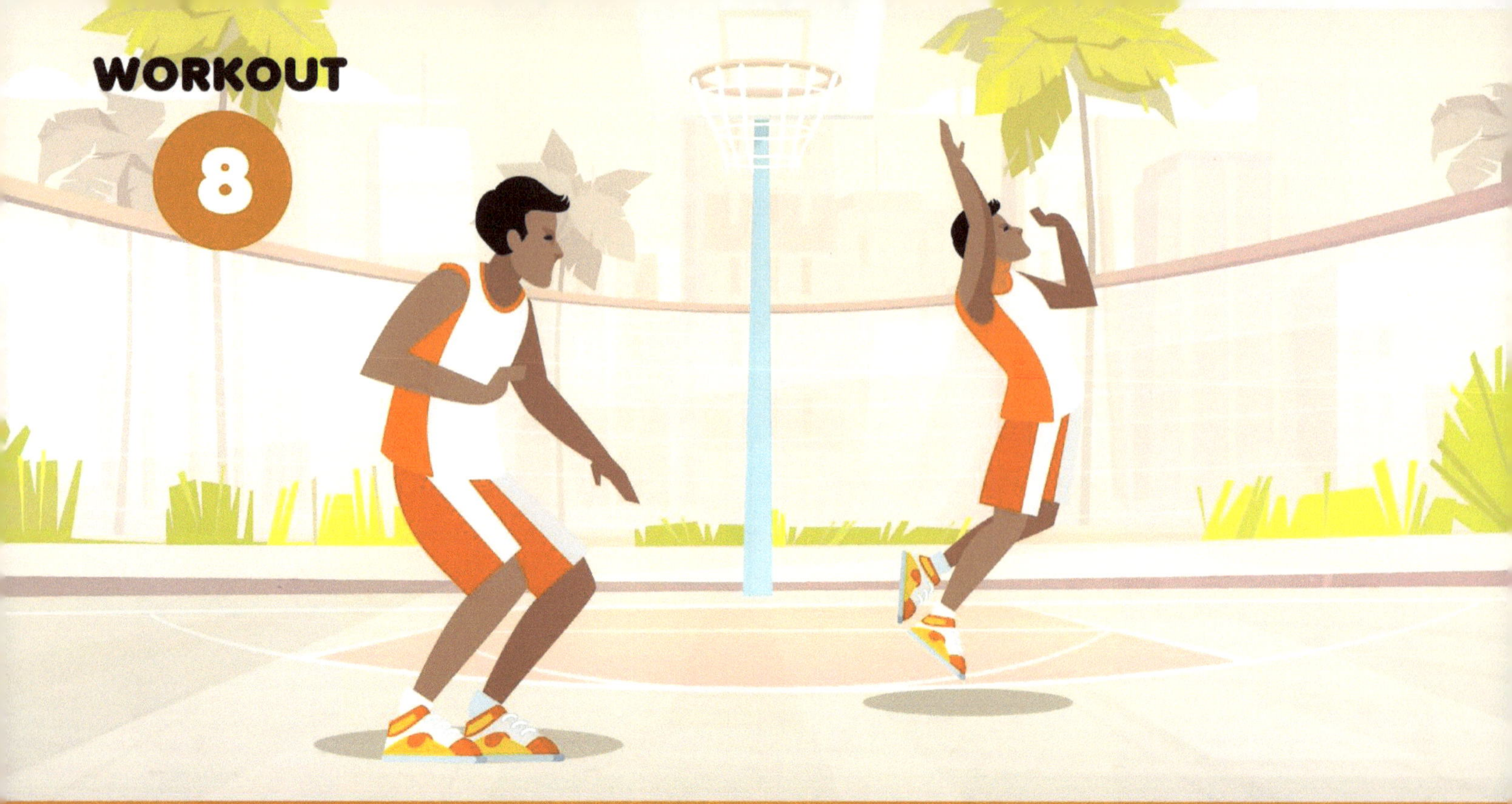

SHUFFLE BASKETBALL SHOTS

HOW LONG?

45

SECS

HOW TO DO IT

In squat position, shuffle to the right a few steps and jump, taking an air basketball shot. Shuffle to the left and repeat.

The only time you'll be shooting threes in every shot.

READY FOR THE NEXT ONE? →

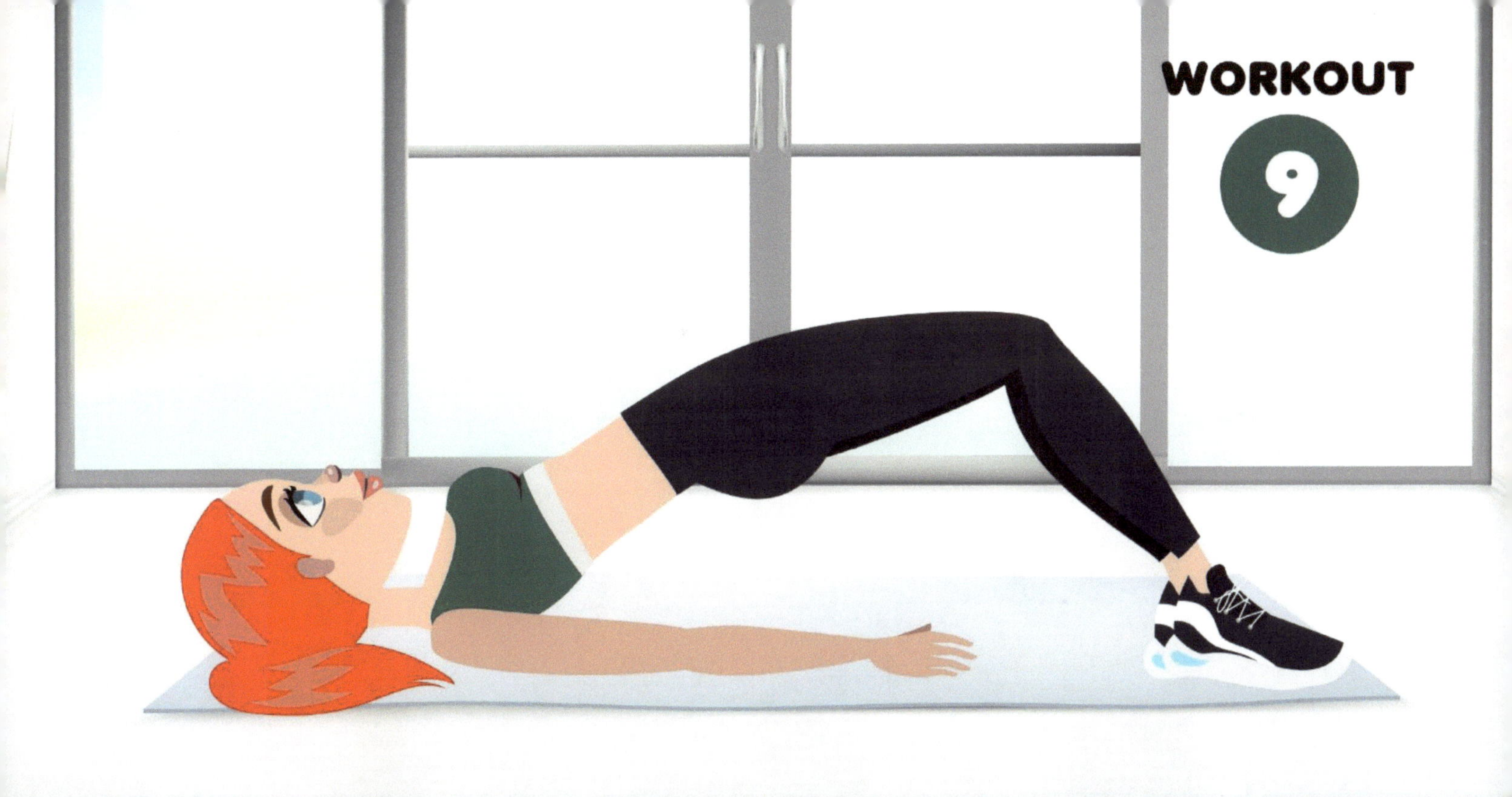

BRIDGE THRUSTS

HOW MANY?

20

HOW TO DO IT

Lying flat on your back, knees bent, thrust your pelvis up towards the sky. Lower back down. Repeat.

To take this up a notch, don't let your bum touch the floor between thrusts.

READY FOR THE NEXT ONE? 

WORKOUT

10

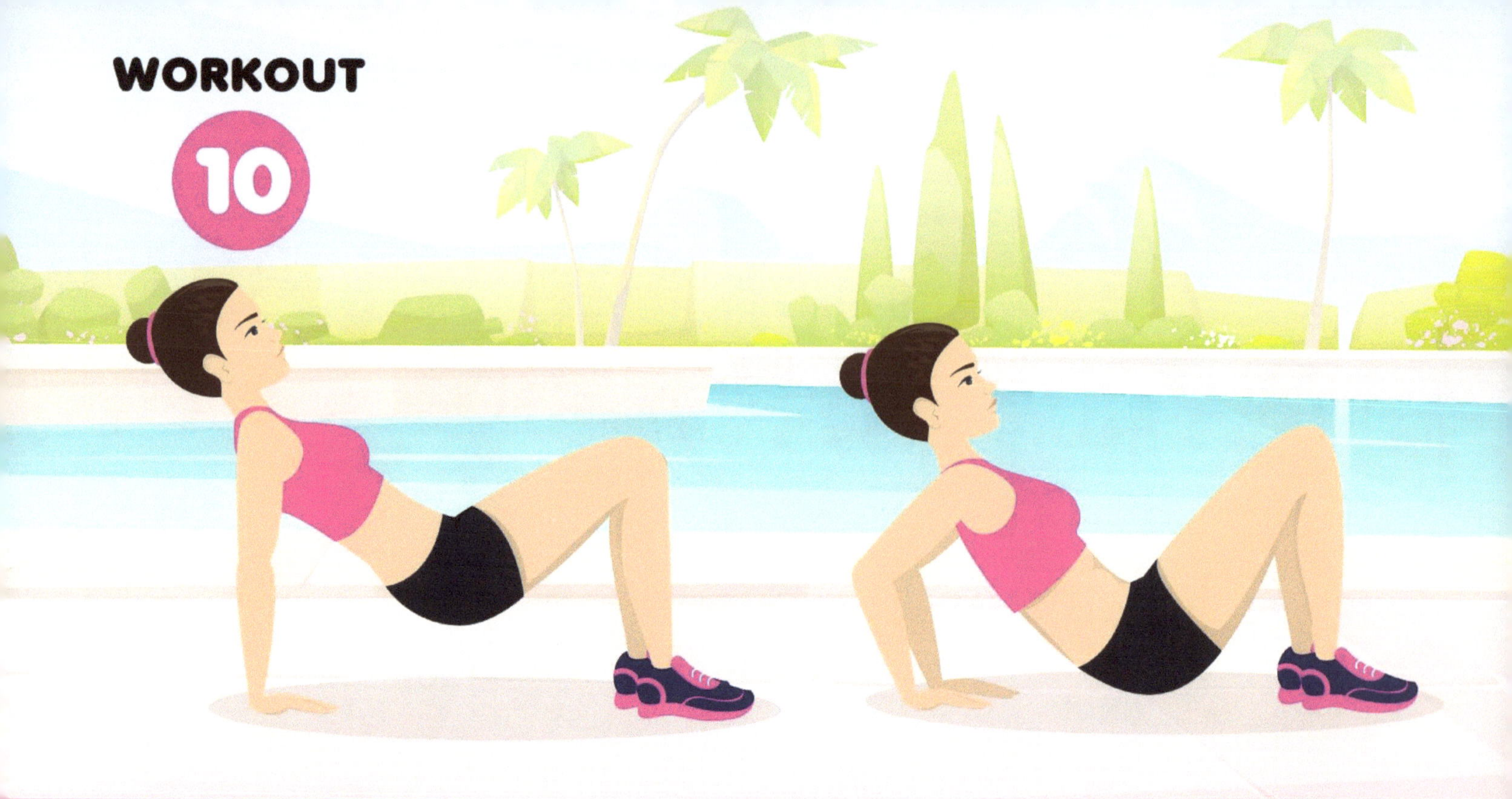

TRICEP DIPS

HOW MANY?

20

HOW TO DO IT

Get into a crab position, flat on the floor or braced on a stair. Lower down by bending your elbows straight behind you. Come back up and repeat.

Mission Flabby Arms Demolition.

READY FOR THE NEXT ONE? →

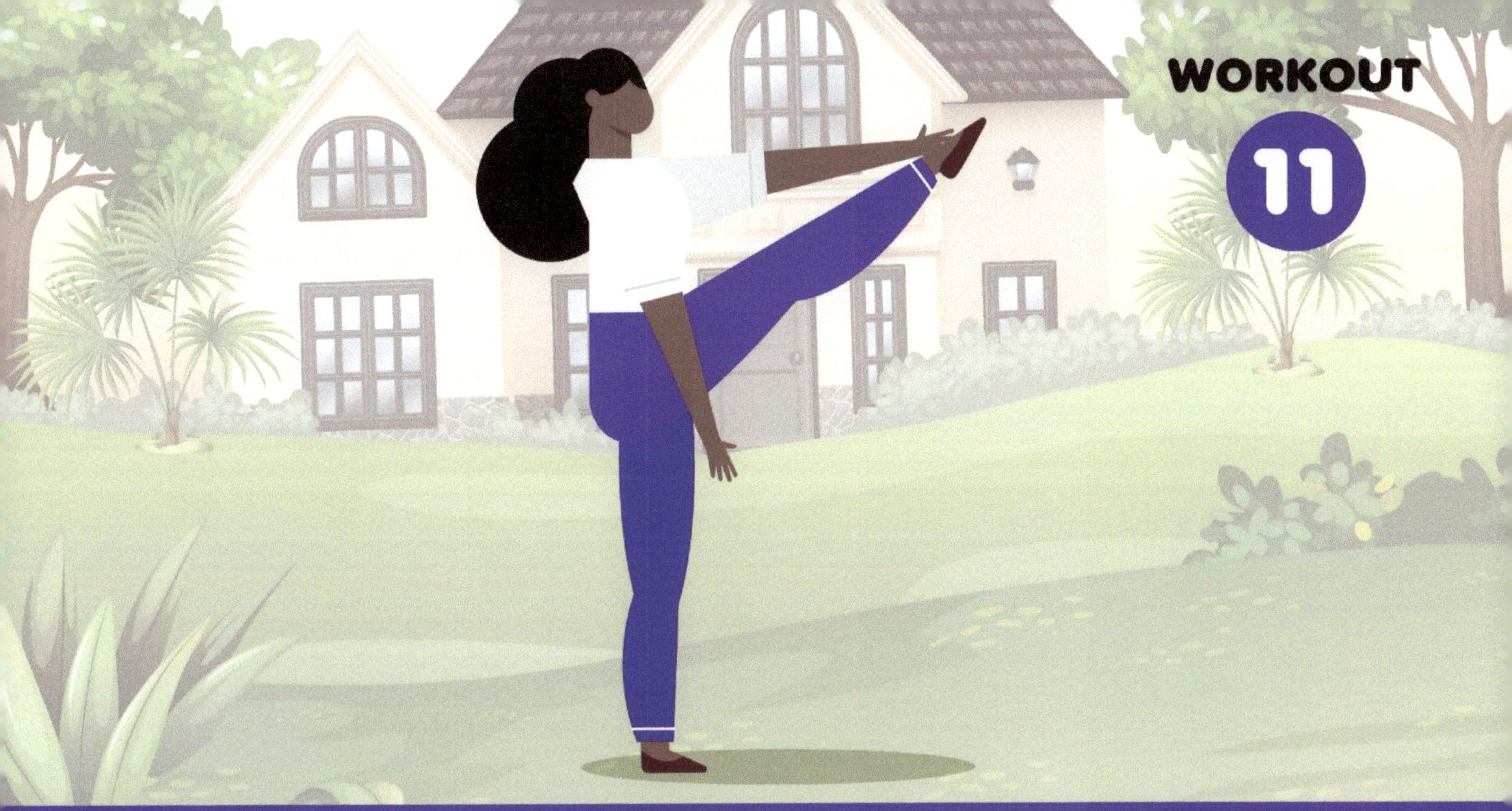

HIGH KICK TOE TOUCH

HOW MANY?

20

TOTAL

HOW TO DO IT

Kick your leg as high as you can, while opposite arm touches the toe (or knee, if you can't reach that far!). Alternate.

Don't worry if you can't touch your toes, flexibility will increase with consistency.

READY FOR THE NEXT ONE? 

WORKOUT

12

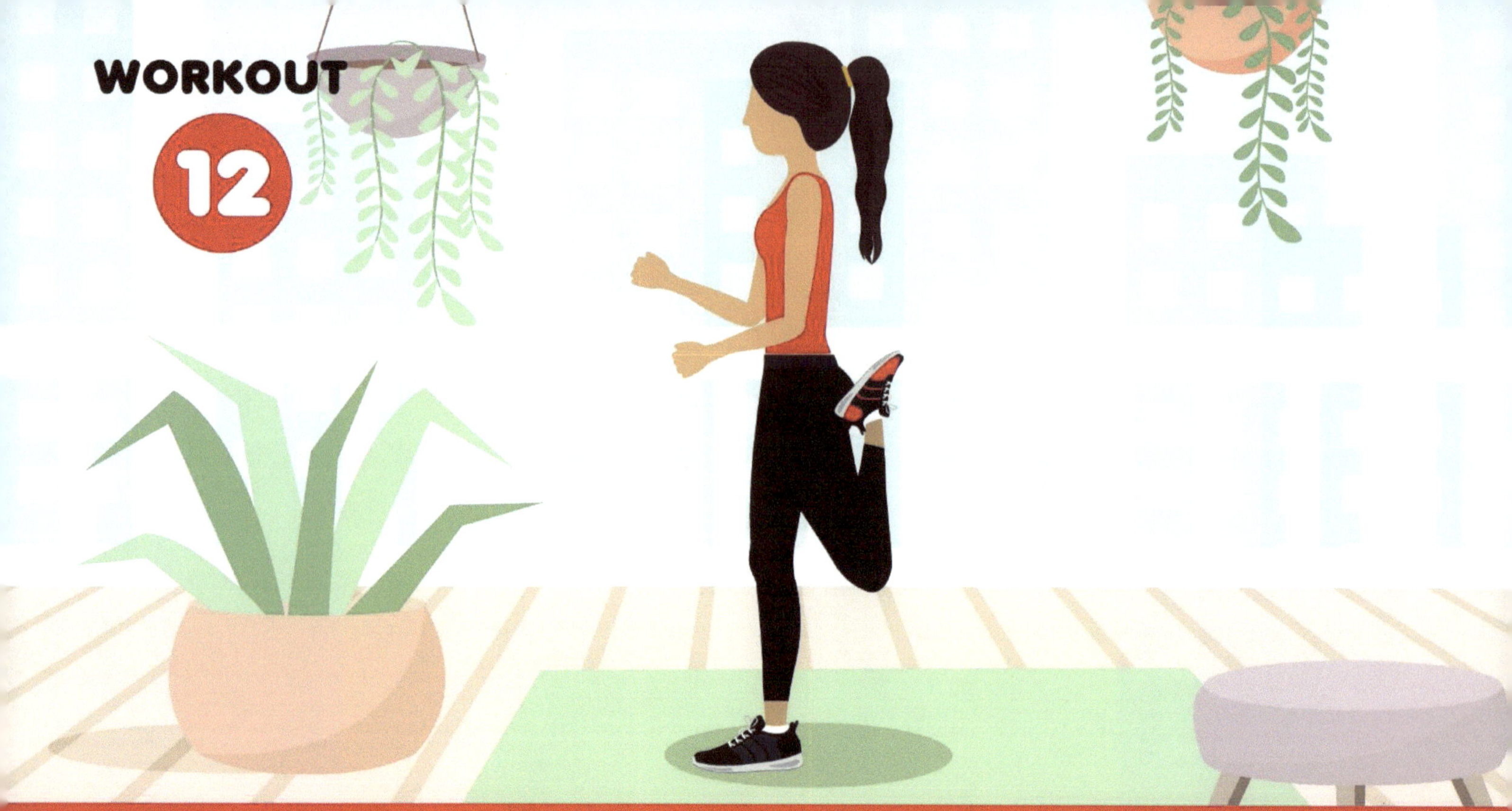

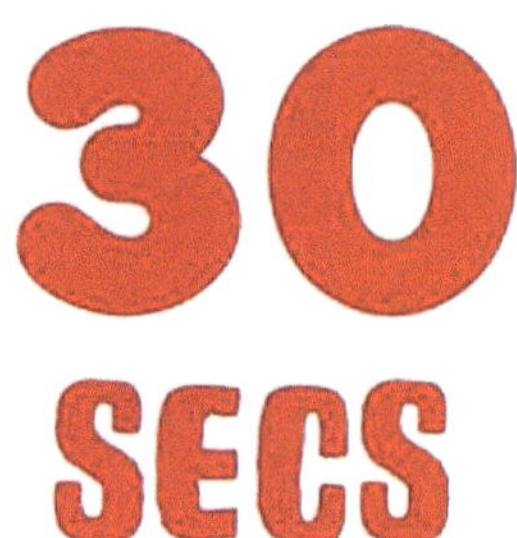

BUTT KICKS

HOW LONG?

30

SECS

HOW TO DO IT

You're jogging on the spot, except your feet are lifting right back to kick yourself in the butt.

It never gets easier. You just get stronger.

READY FOR THE NEXT ONE?

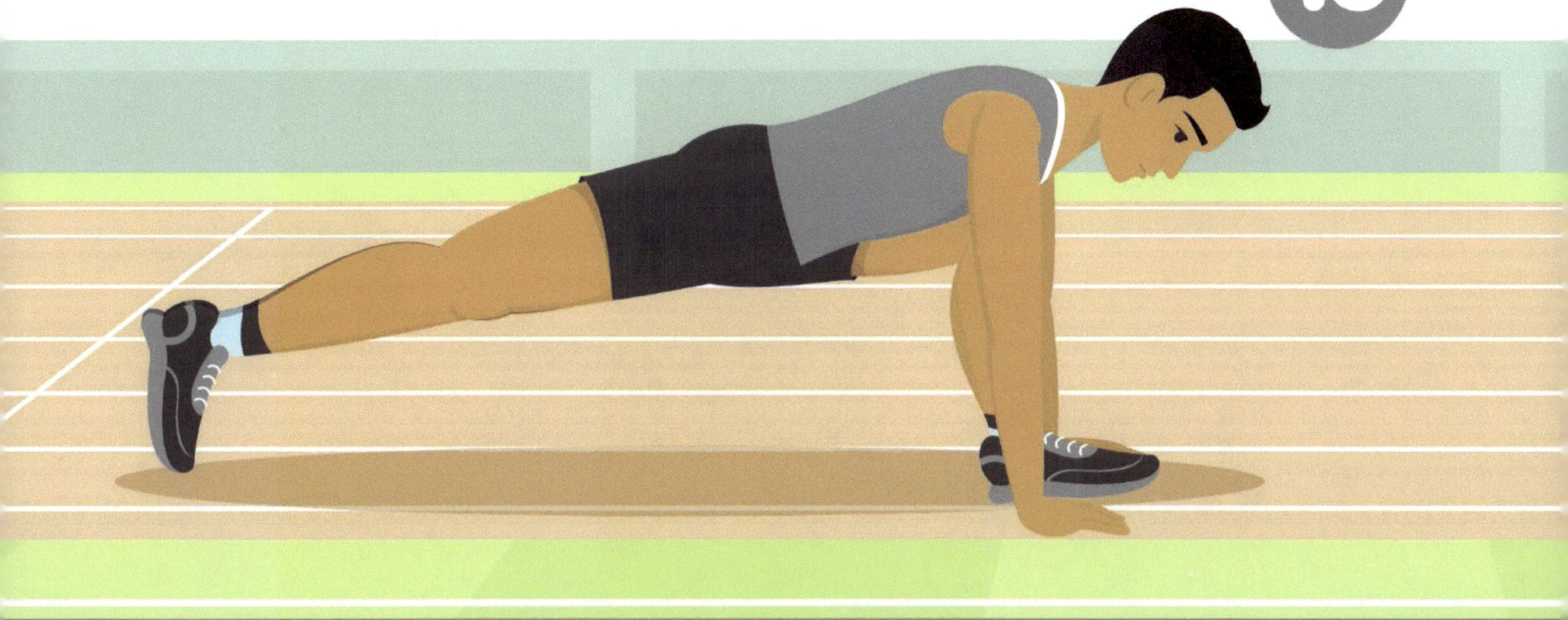

RUNNER'S STRETCH

HOW LONG?

15 SECS

EACH SIDE

HOW TO DO IT

Starting on the floor, lean your chest against a bent knee and stretch the opposite leg straight behind you. Put the weight in your front heel for the stretch.

The stretch that keeps your hamstrings beautiful.

READY FOR THE NEXT ONE? 

WORKOUT

14

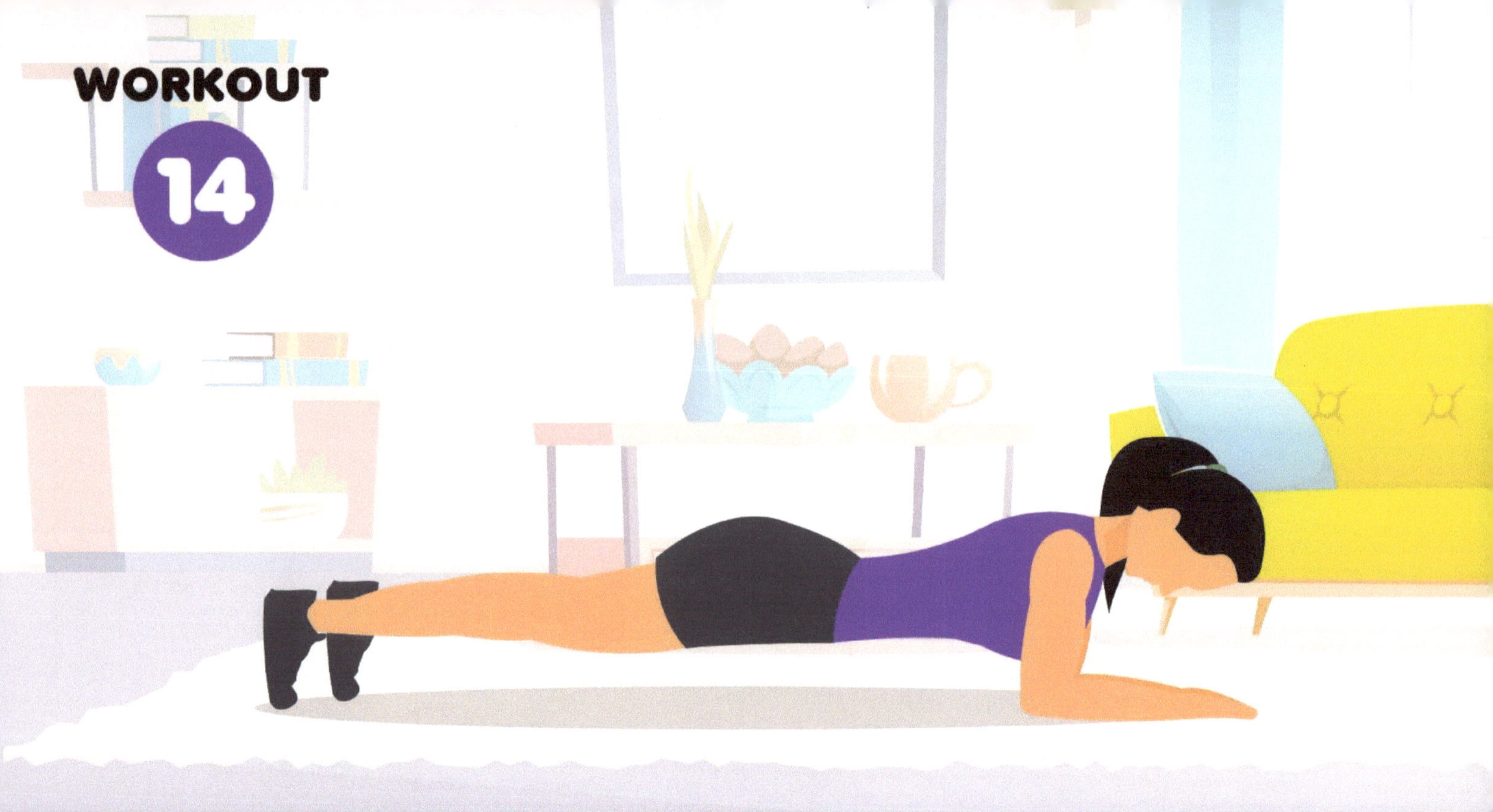

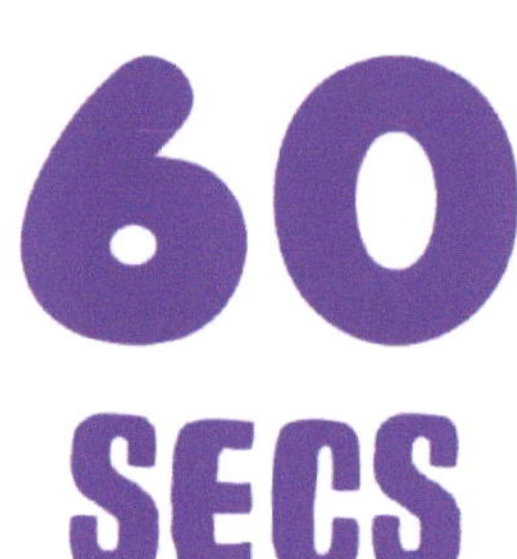

PLANK

HOW LONG?

60 SECS

HOW TO DO IT

Hold your body in a pushup position, resting your forearms or hands on the ground.

A minute goes by really fast . . . until you're planking.

READY FOR THE NEXT ONE?

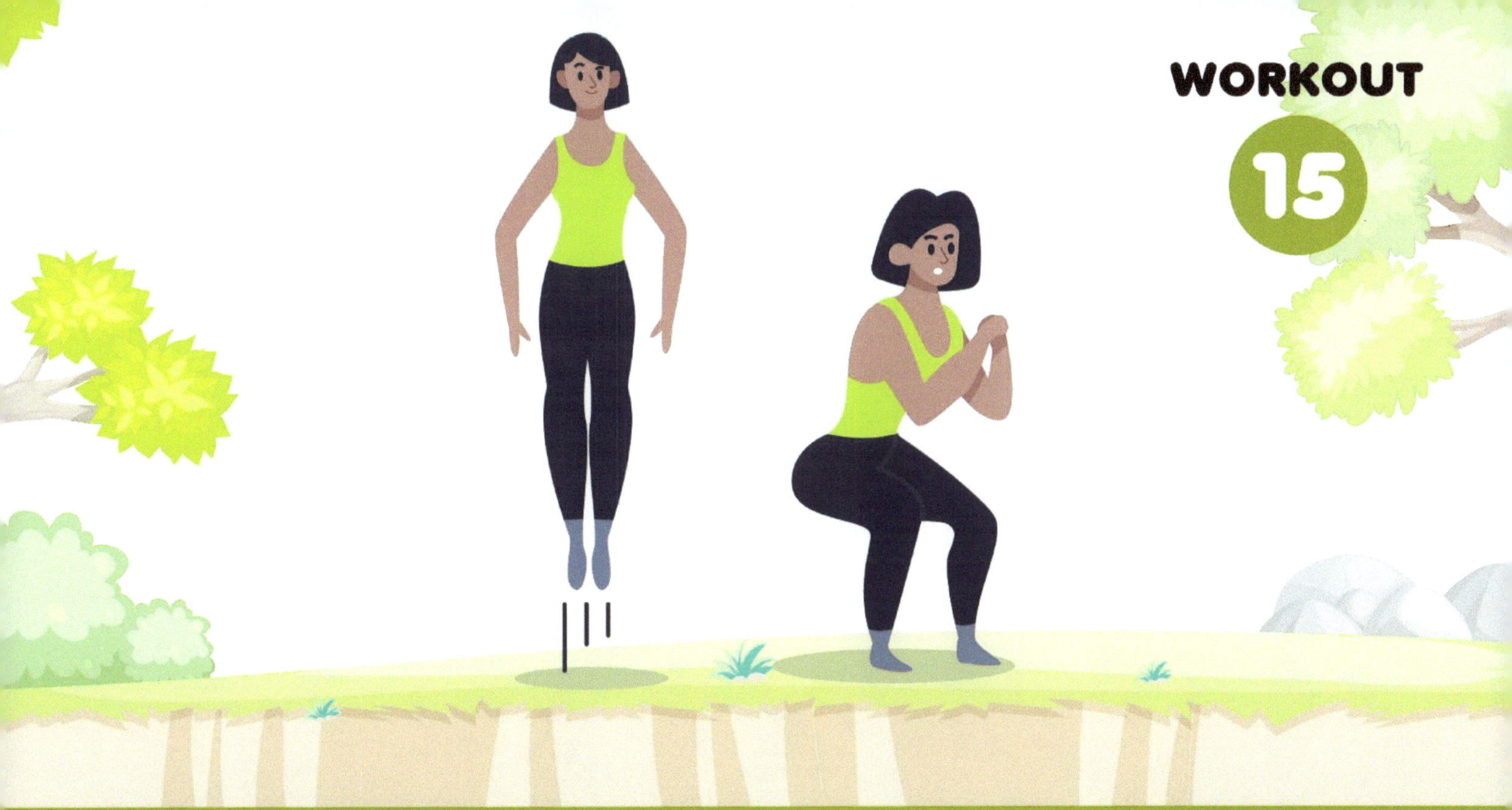

JUMP SQUATS

HOW MANY?

15

HOW TO DO IT

Jump and landing on soft knees, go right into a squat. After your squat, launch right into your jump again.

Shake your legs out after this one or you'll be walking like Lego men.

READY FOR THE NEXT ONE? 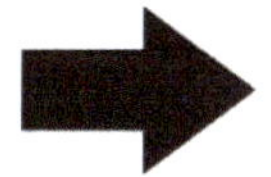

WORKOUT

16

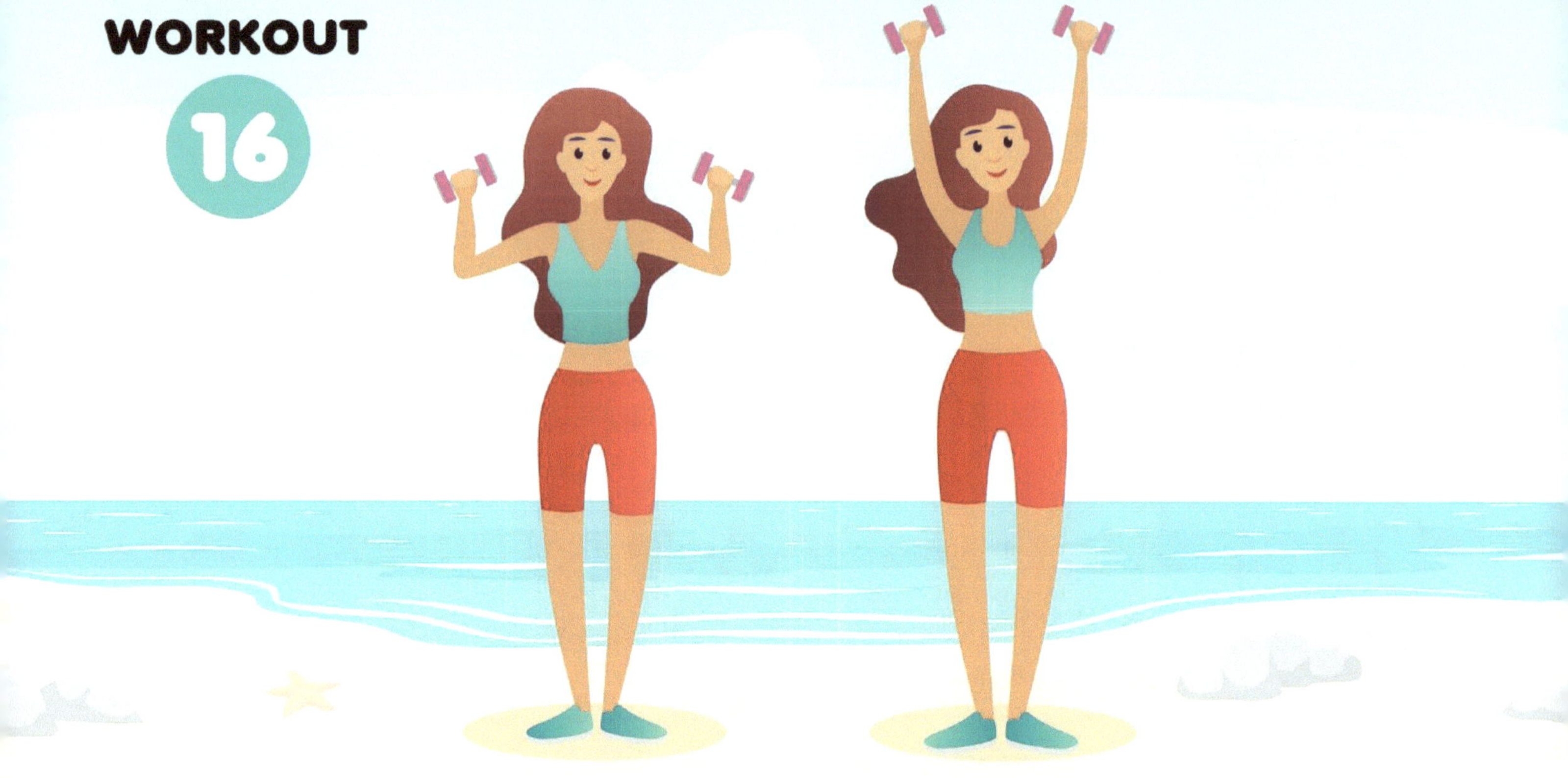

SHOULDER PRESS

HOW MANY?

20

HOW TO DO IT

Using dumbbells, soup cans or whatever you have, press your arms from a U position, up to the sky and back down.

Make it burn, so that it will hurt to put on a shirt tomorrow.

READY FOR THE NEXT ONE? →

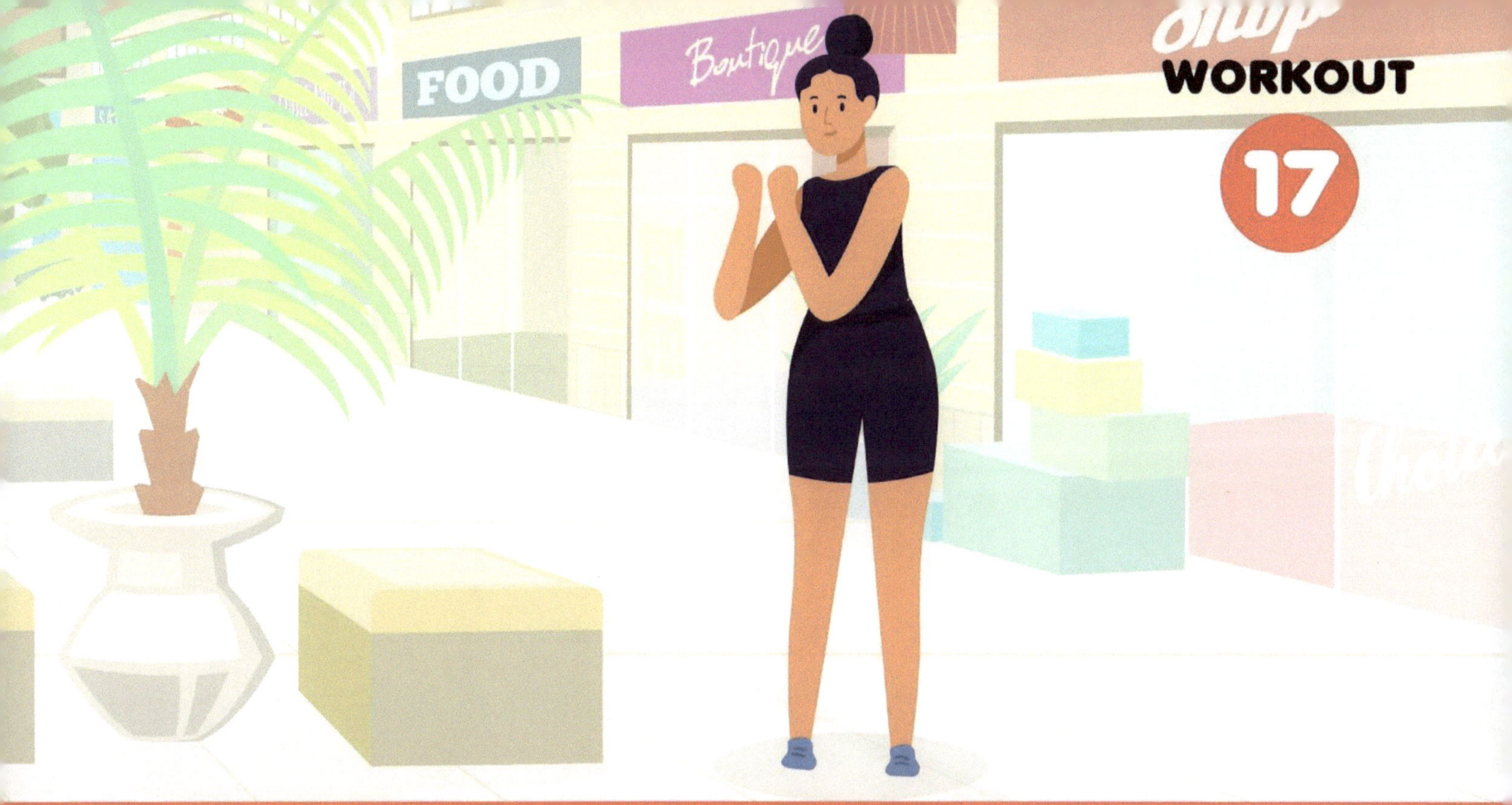

STANDING CRUNCHES

HOW MANY?

35

HOW TO DO IT

Standing, crouch slightly, letting your abs do the work to bend you. Arms can be up or down - abs are doing the work here!

Don't hold your breath for this one!

READY FOR THE NEXT ONE? 

WORKOUT 18

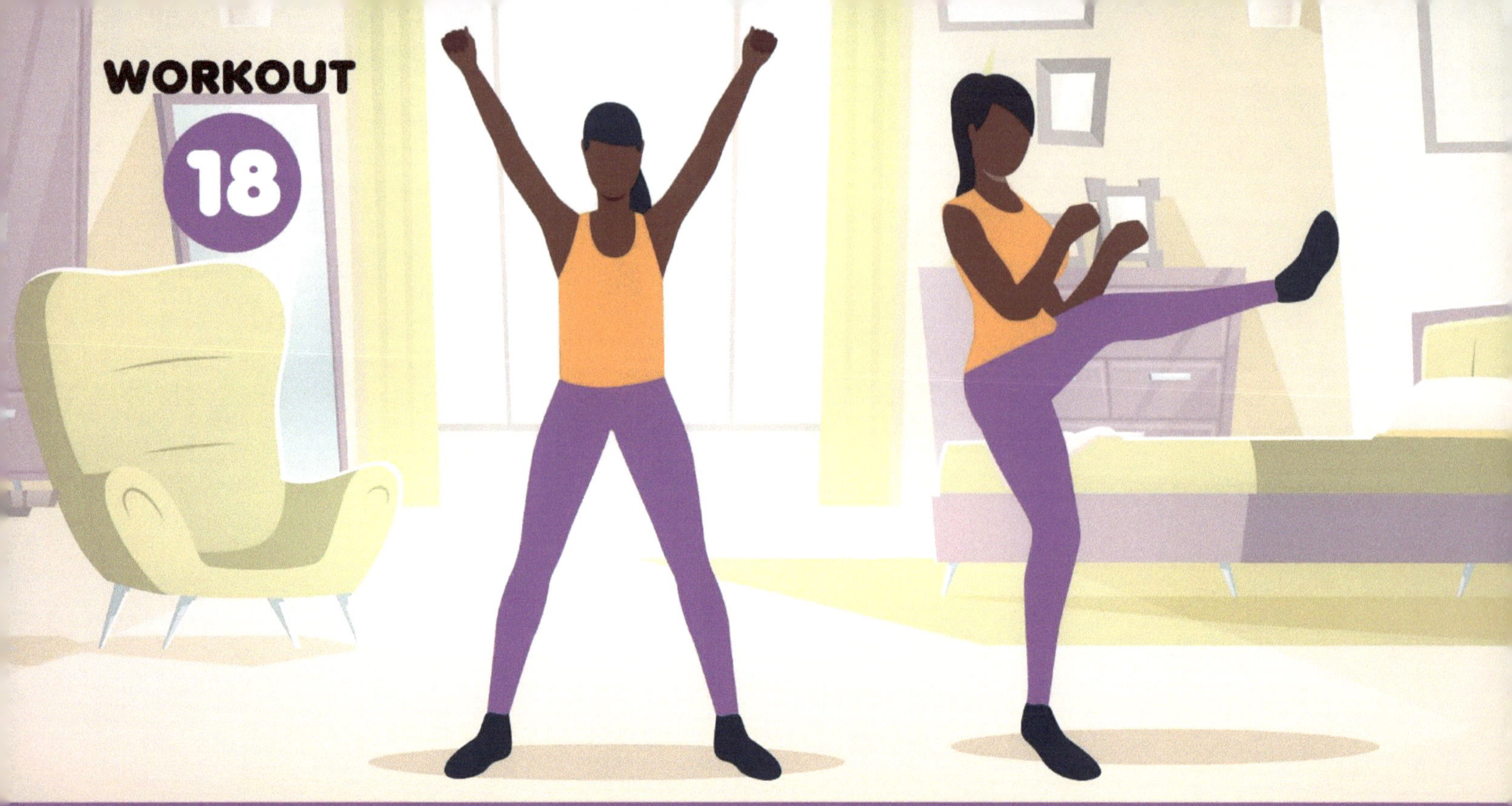

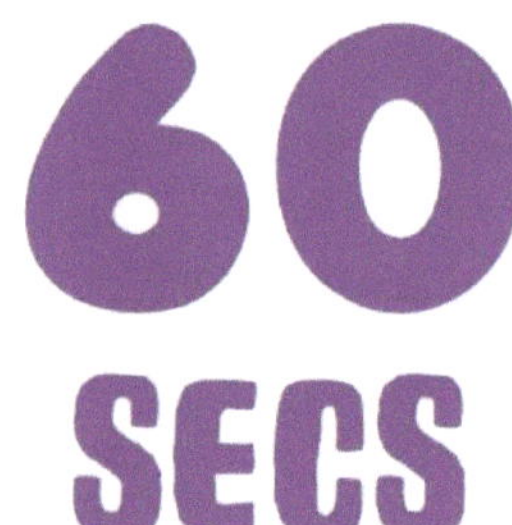

JACK WITH KICK

HOW LONG?

60 SECS

HOW TO DO IT

Do a jumping jack, then do a front kick with one leg. Do another jack, then kick with other leg. Keep alternating.

Twinkle, twinkle, little star,
jumping jack, then kick it hard

READY FOR THE NEXT ONE?

WORKOUT

19

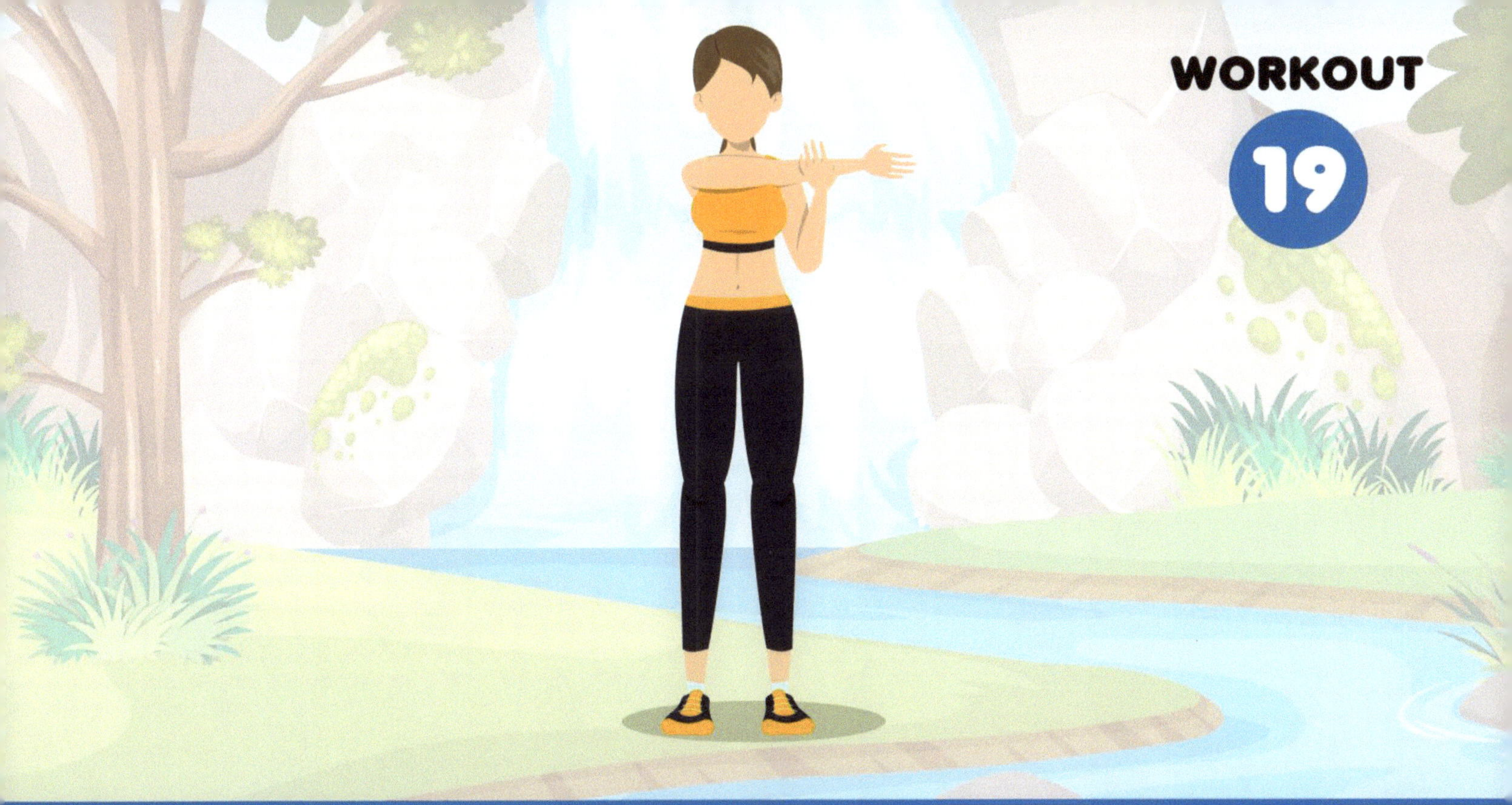

SHOULDER STRETCH

HOW MANY?

15 SECS

EACH SIDE

HOW TO DO IT

Cross your arm across your body. Hold your elbow for the duration of the stretch.

Pull off to the side of the road, if you need a shoulder to cry on. This is a tear-free zone.

READY FOR THE NEXT ONE?

WORKOUT

20

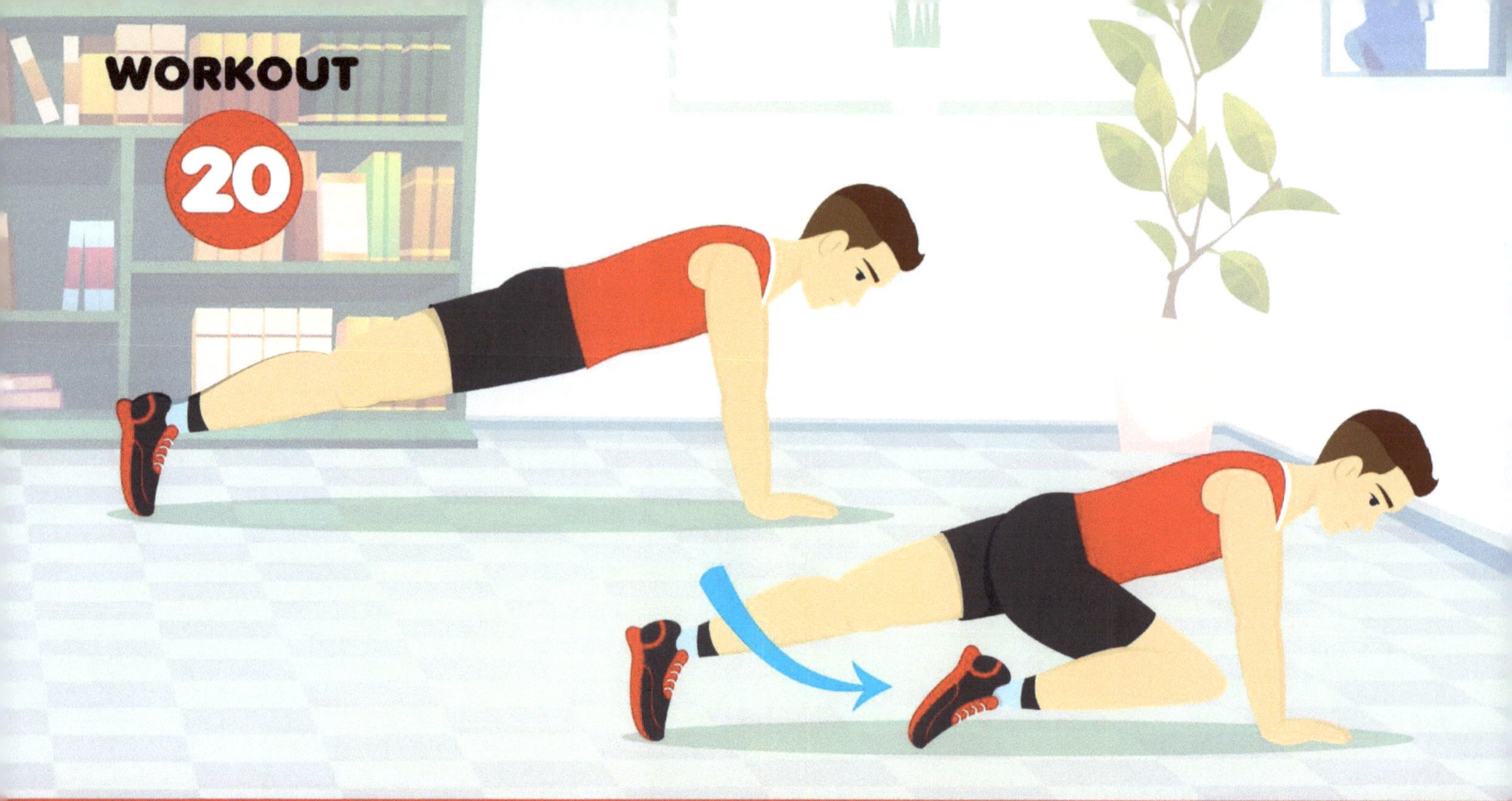

MOUNTAIN CLIMBERS

HOW LONG?

30

SECS

HOW TO DO IT

Get in plank position. Lift one knee up to your chest, back to plank, then the other knee to chest. Run in this position.

This is probably the closest anyone is going to get you to go mountain climbing.

READY FOR THE NEXT ONE?

WORKOUT

21

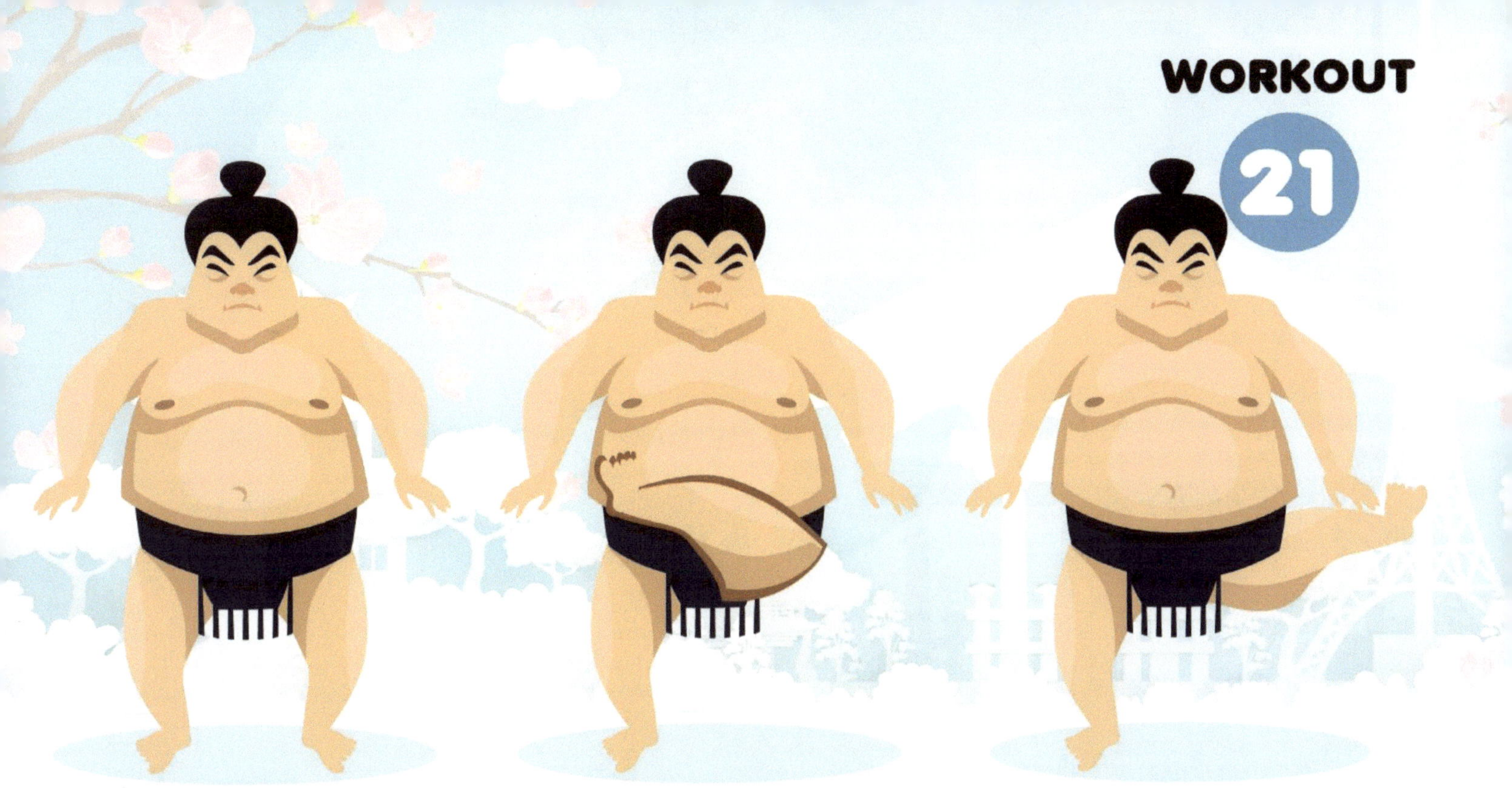

SUMO ROUNDKICKS

HOW MANY?

20

TOTAL

HOW TO DO IT

Slowly do a roundkick. Sweep each leg in a circular round motion through the air in front of you. Alternate.

Also known as a Crescent Kick. Your thighs will need a lazy day tomorrow after this.

READY FOR THE NEXT ONE? →

WORKOUT

22

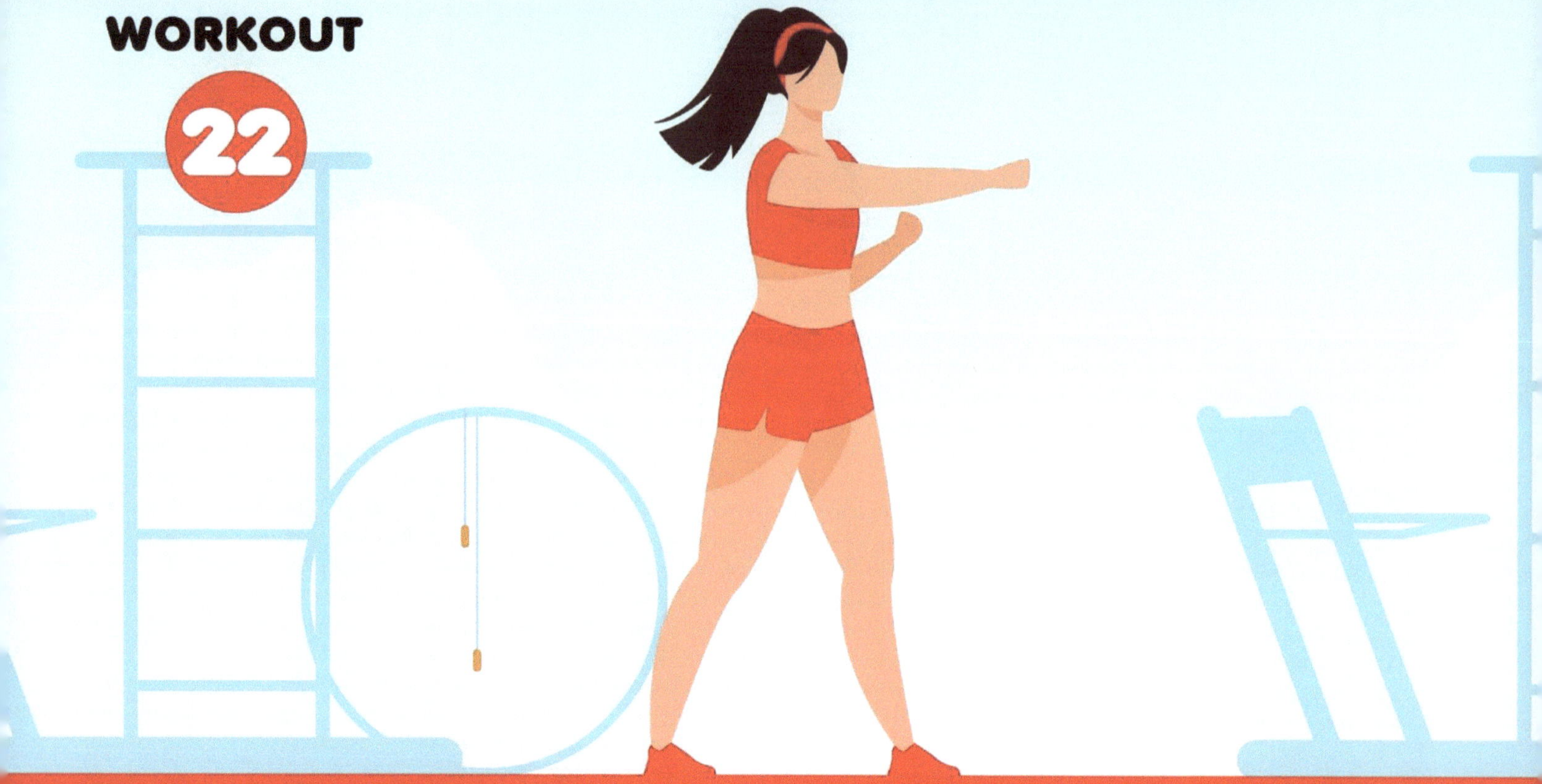

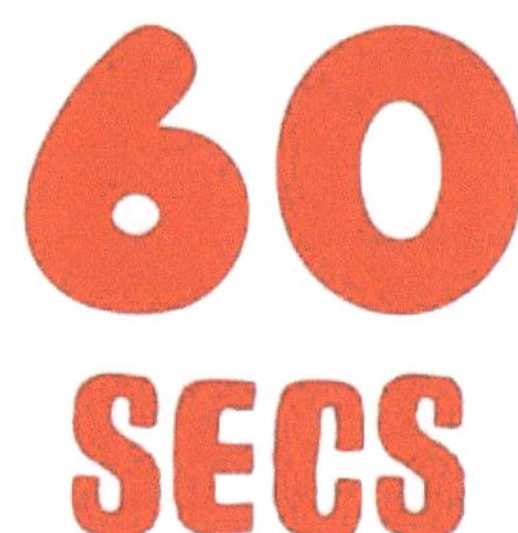

PUNCHES

HOW LONG?

60

SECS

HOW TO DO IT

You can punch slow with force, for strength training or fast and quick, for cardio.

Punch like you're beating up your arm fat and you'll knock it down in no time.

READY FOR THE NEXT ONE? ➡

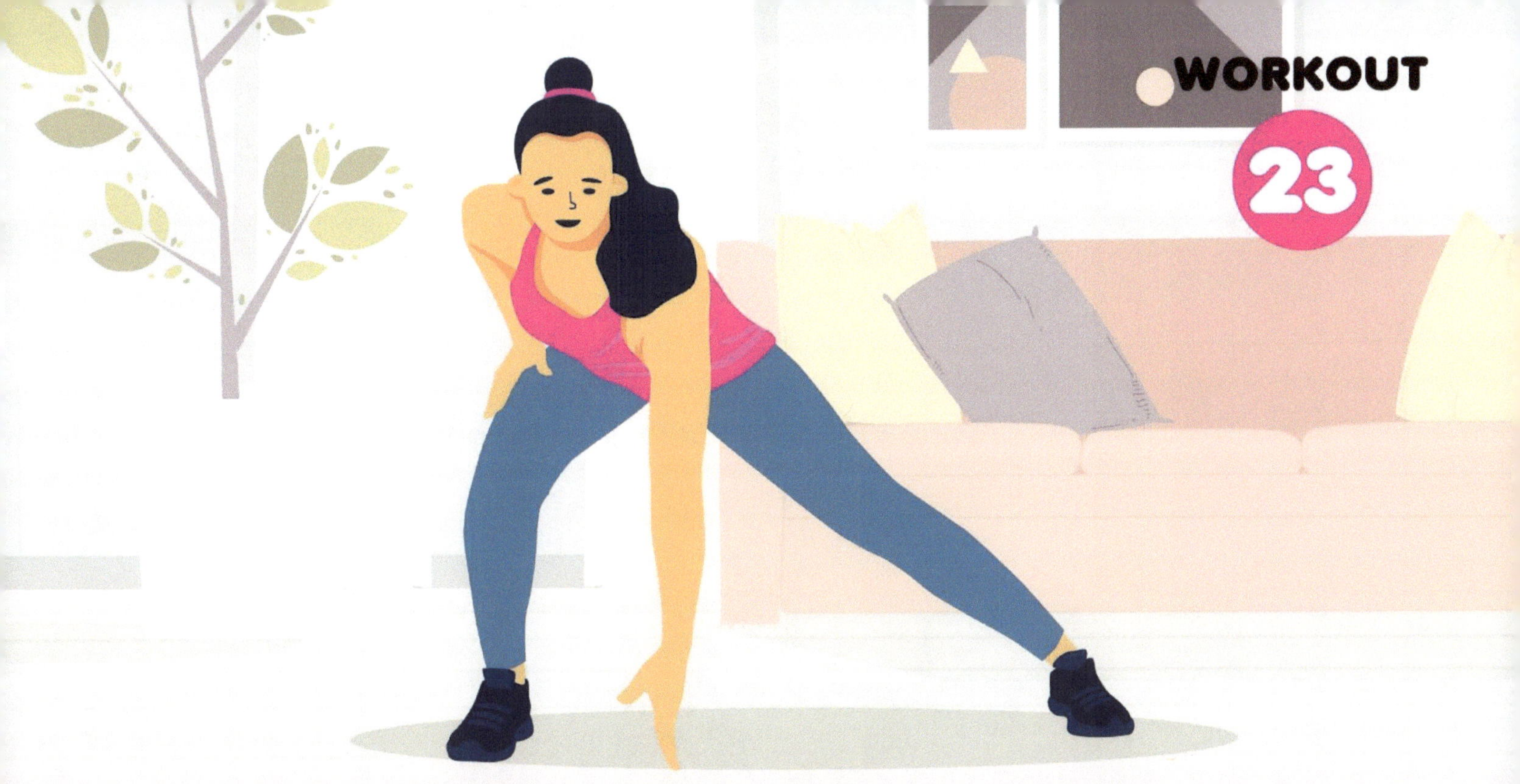

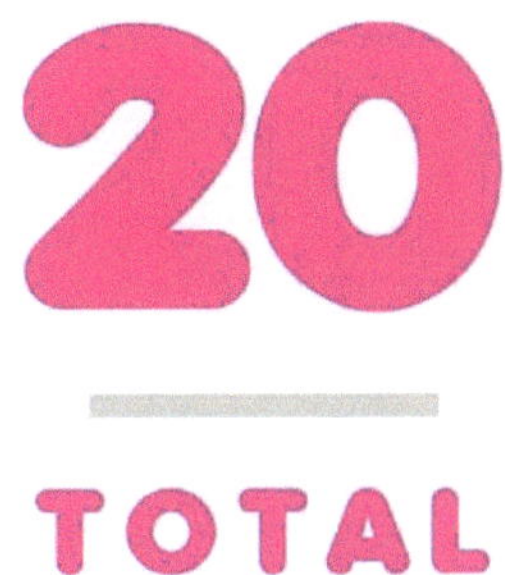

SIDE LUNGE FLOOR TOUCH

HOW MANY?

20

TOTAL

HOW TO DO IT

Lunge to the side, then touch the floor with opposite arm. Stand to center. Alternate.

Don't wish for a good body, work for it.

READY FOR THE NEXT ONE? 

WORKOUT

24

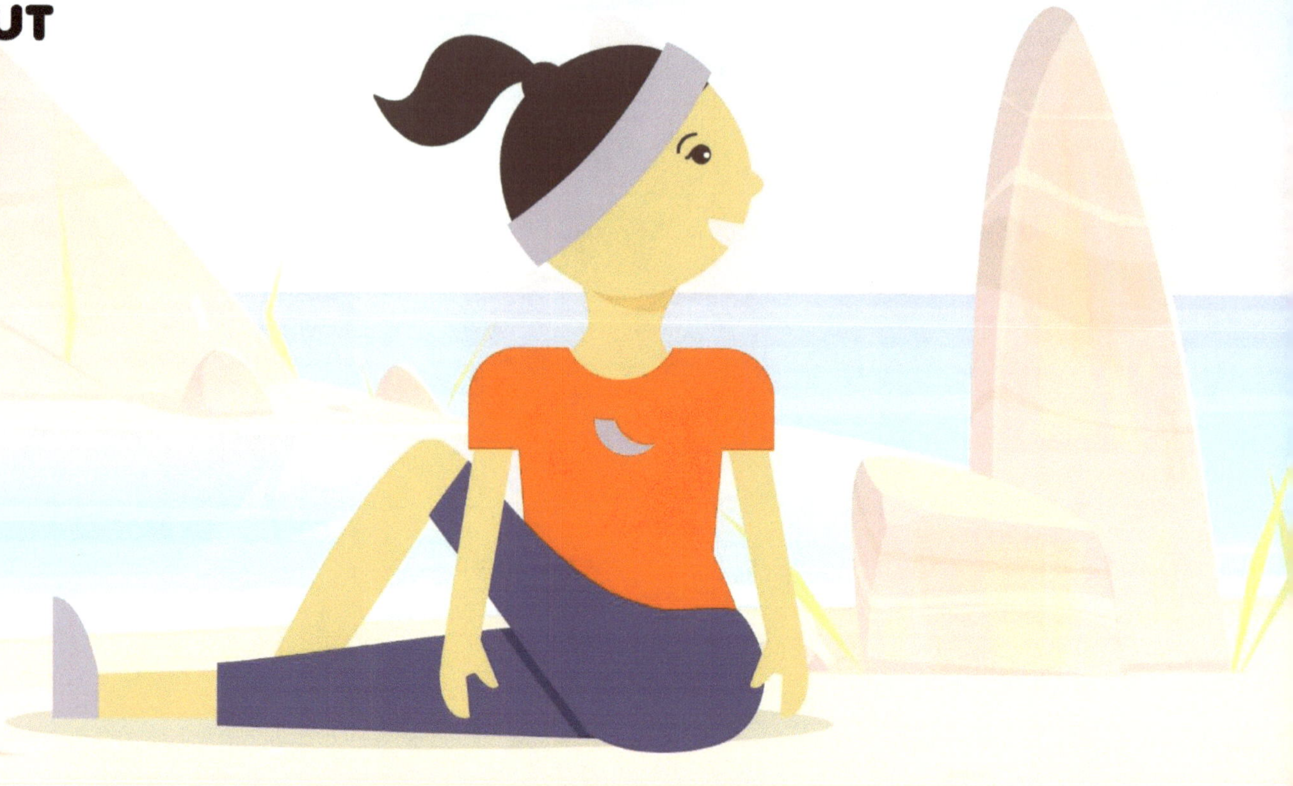

CROSS LEG TWIST STRETCH

HOW LONG?

15 SECS

EACH SIDE

HOW TO DO IT

Sitting up with legs flat, cross a bent leg over the other. Look over the shoulder of the bent knee, arm pressed against bent leg. Hold.

Stretches help flexibility. Flexibility turbo boosts workouts. Workouts get results.

READY FOR THE NEXT ONE?

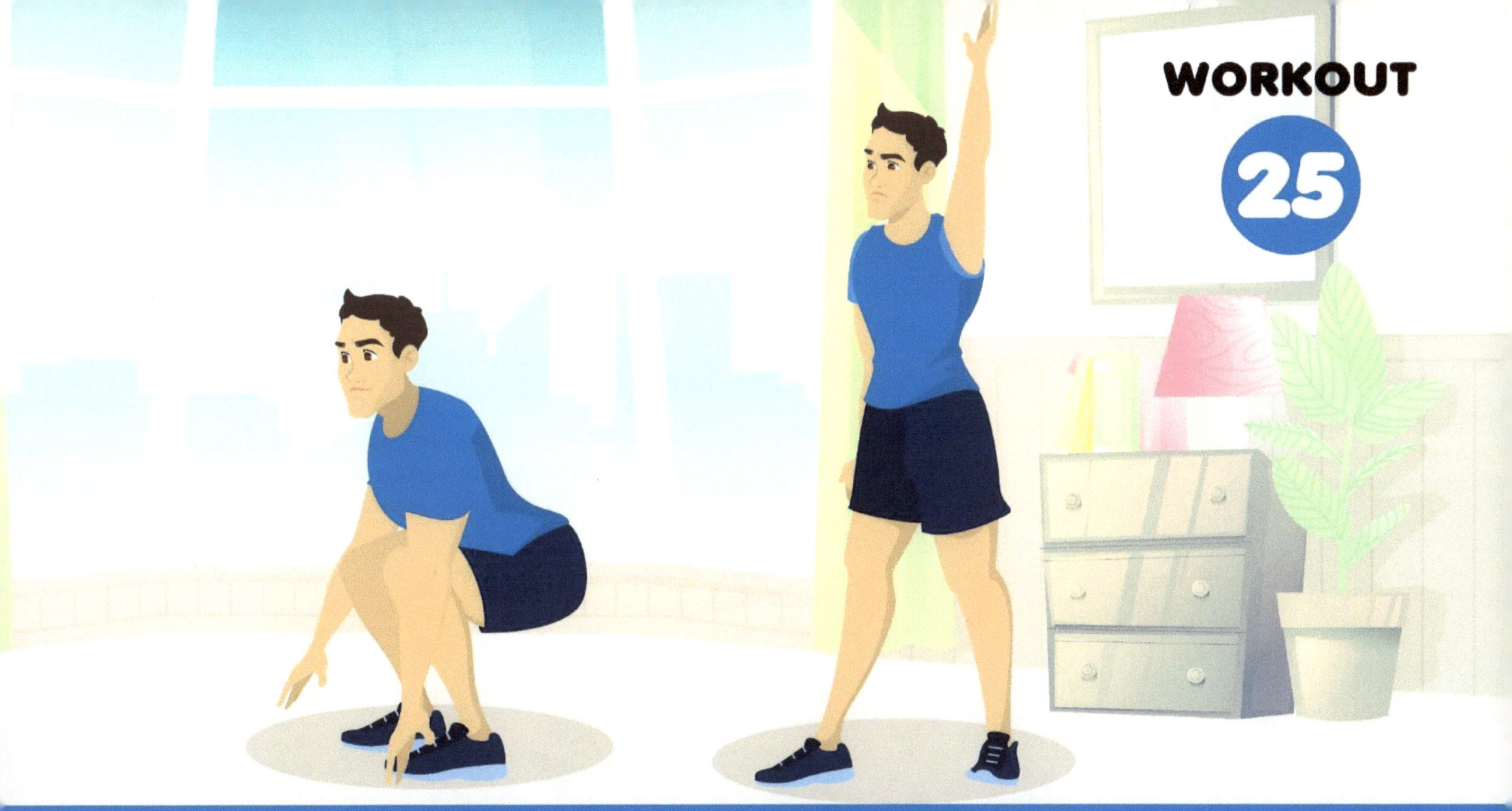

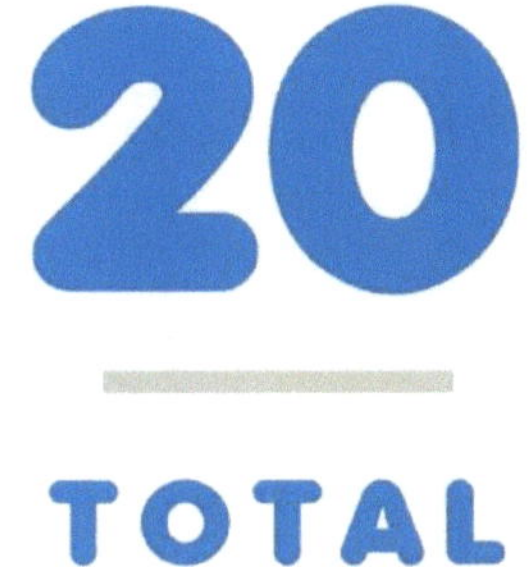

SQUAT FLOOR TO SKY

HOW MANY?

20
TOTAL

HOW TO DO IT

Squat down, touch the floor, then stand and raise that same arm and reach the sky. Alternate. Dumbbells optional.

Life has ups and downs, but today we'll call it "squats".

READY FOR THE NEXT ONE? 

WORKOUT

26

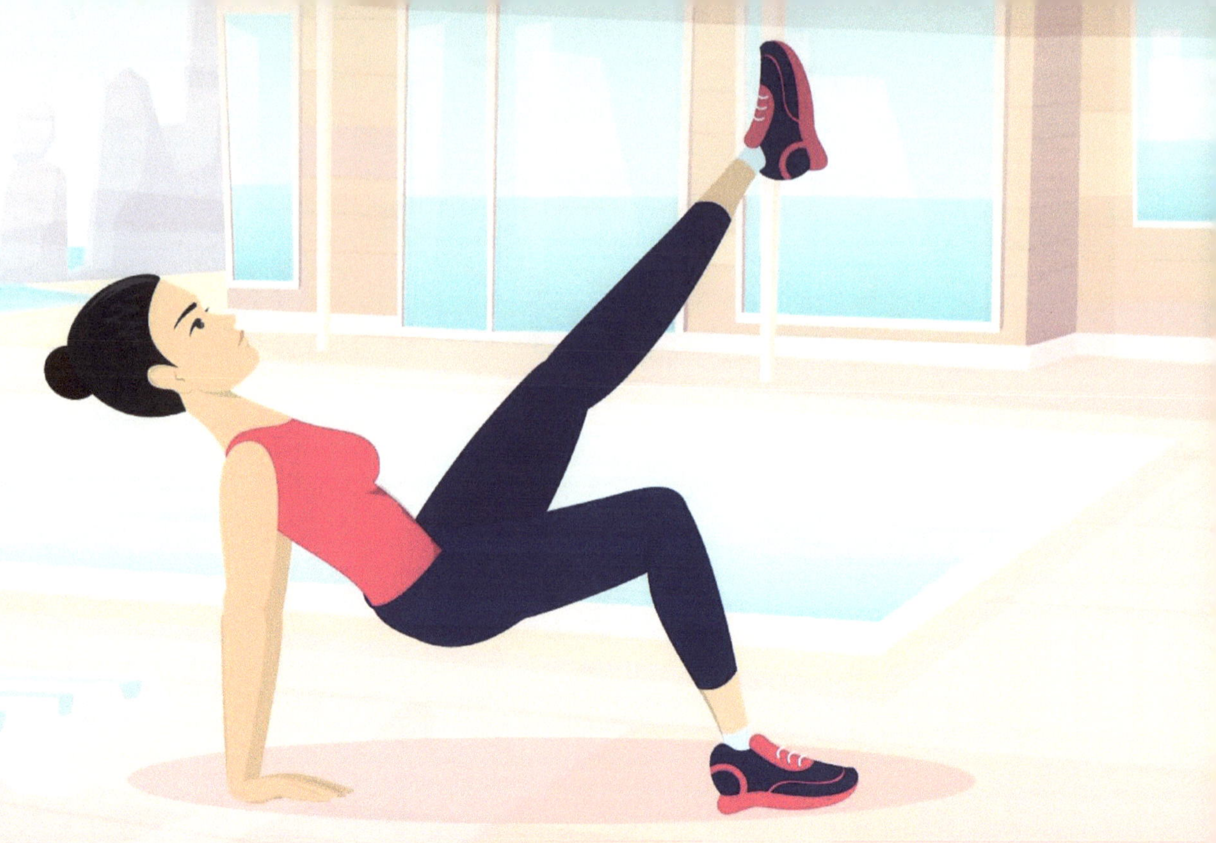

CRAB KICKS

HOW LONG?

45

SECS

HOW TO DO IT

Crab position - hands flat, knees bent, feet flat on ground. Lift your bum slightly off the ground then rotate kicking each leg high in the air.

The only time it's okay to be crabby.

READY FOR THE NEXT ONE? ➡

WORKOUT

27

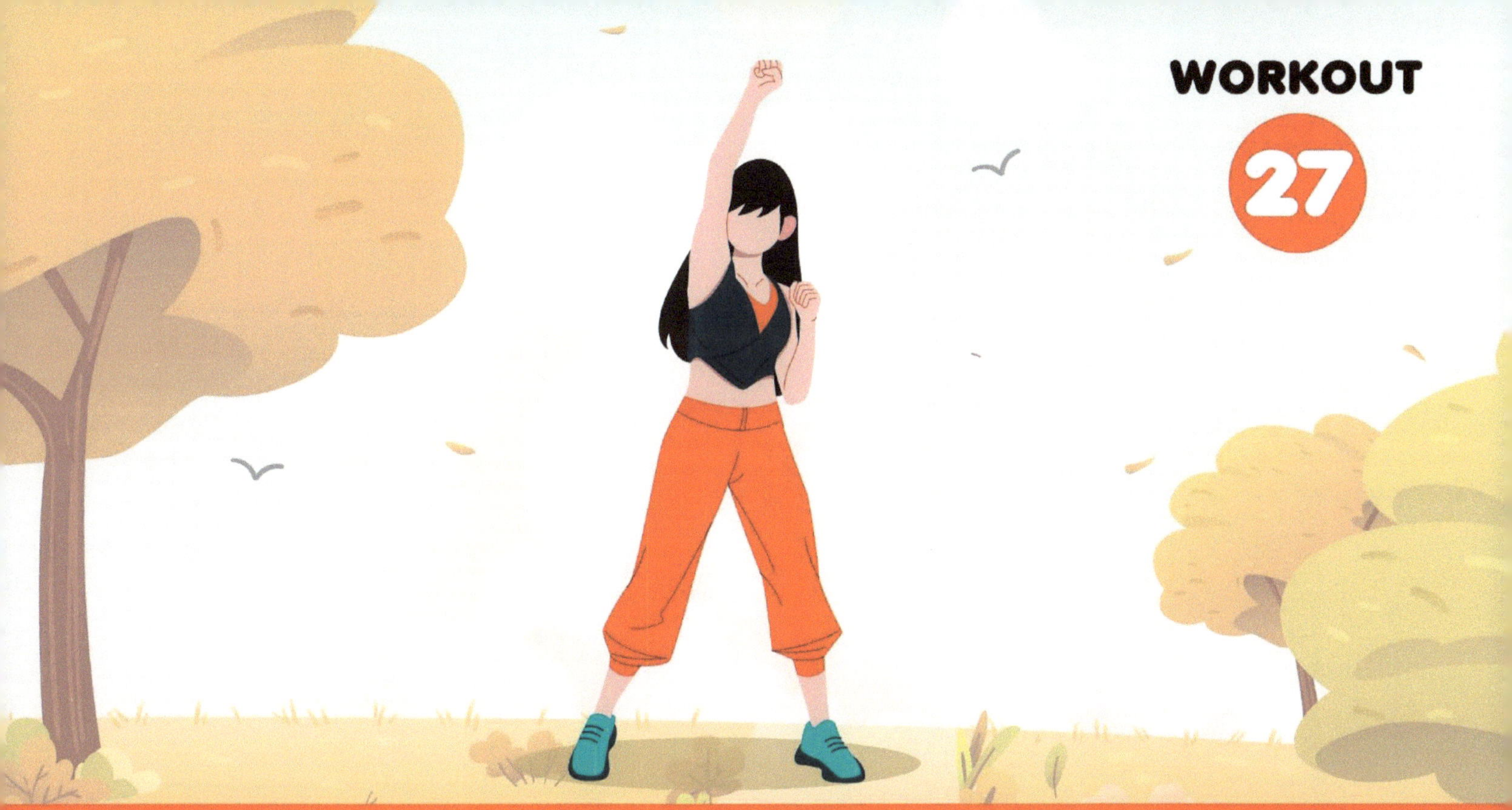

SKY PUNCHES

HOW LONG?

45

SECS

HOW TO DO IT

Alternating arms, punch each fist up to the sky. Don't pause or stop until your time is up.

The moment you're hoping you've purchased an effective deodorant.

READY FOR THE NEXT ONE? ➡

WORKOUT

28

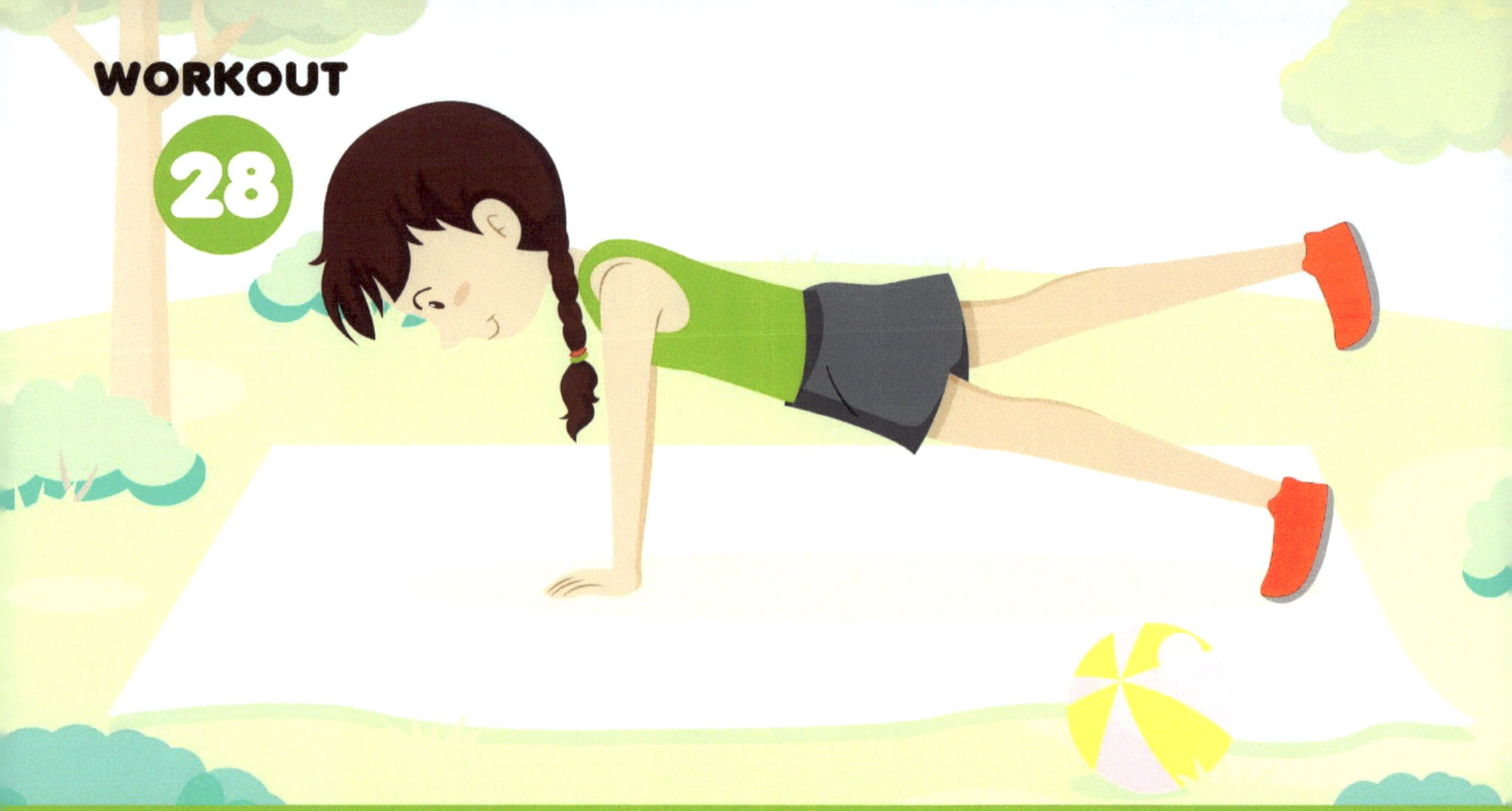

LEG LIFTS IN PLANK

HOW MANY?

20

TOTAL

HOW TO DO IT

Get into plank position, and alternate raising each leg as high as you can lift it.

Excuses don't kill fat - exercises do.

READY FOR THE NEXT ONE? →

WORKOUT

29

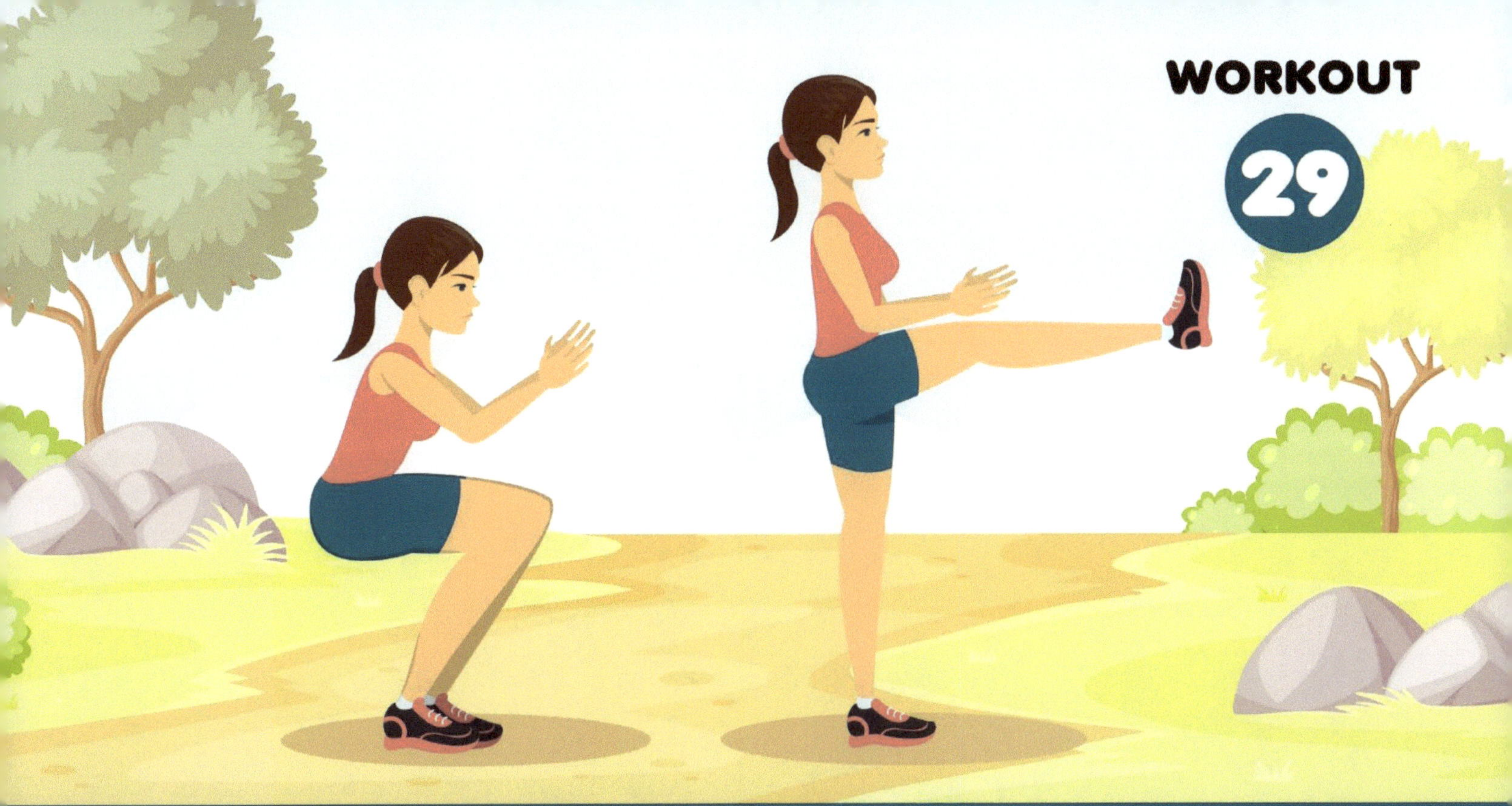

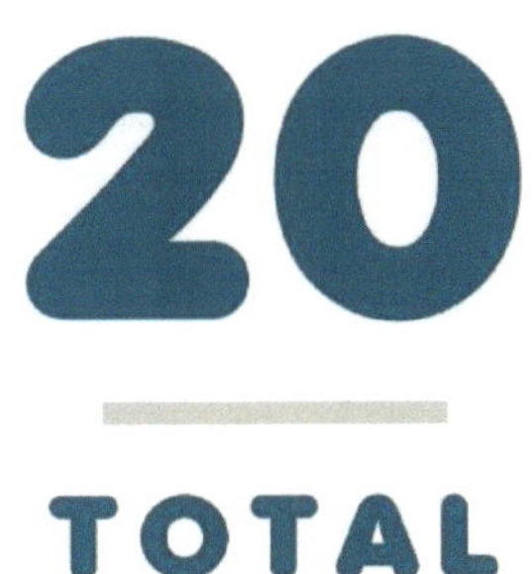

SQUAT WITH KICKS

HOW MANY?

20

TOTAL

HOW TO DO IT

Squat, stand, right leg kick.
Squat, stand, left leg kick.

Kick with your heels, not your knees.
You'll need those when you get older.

READY FOR THE NEXT ONE? →

WORKOUT

30

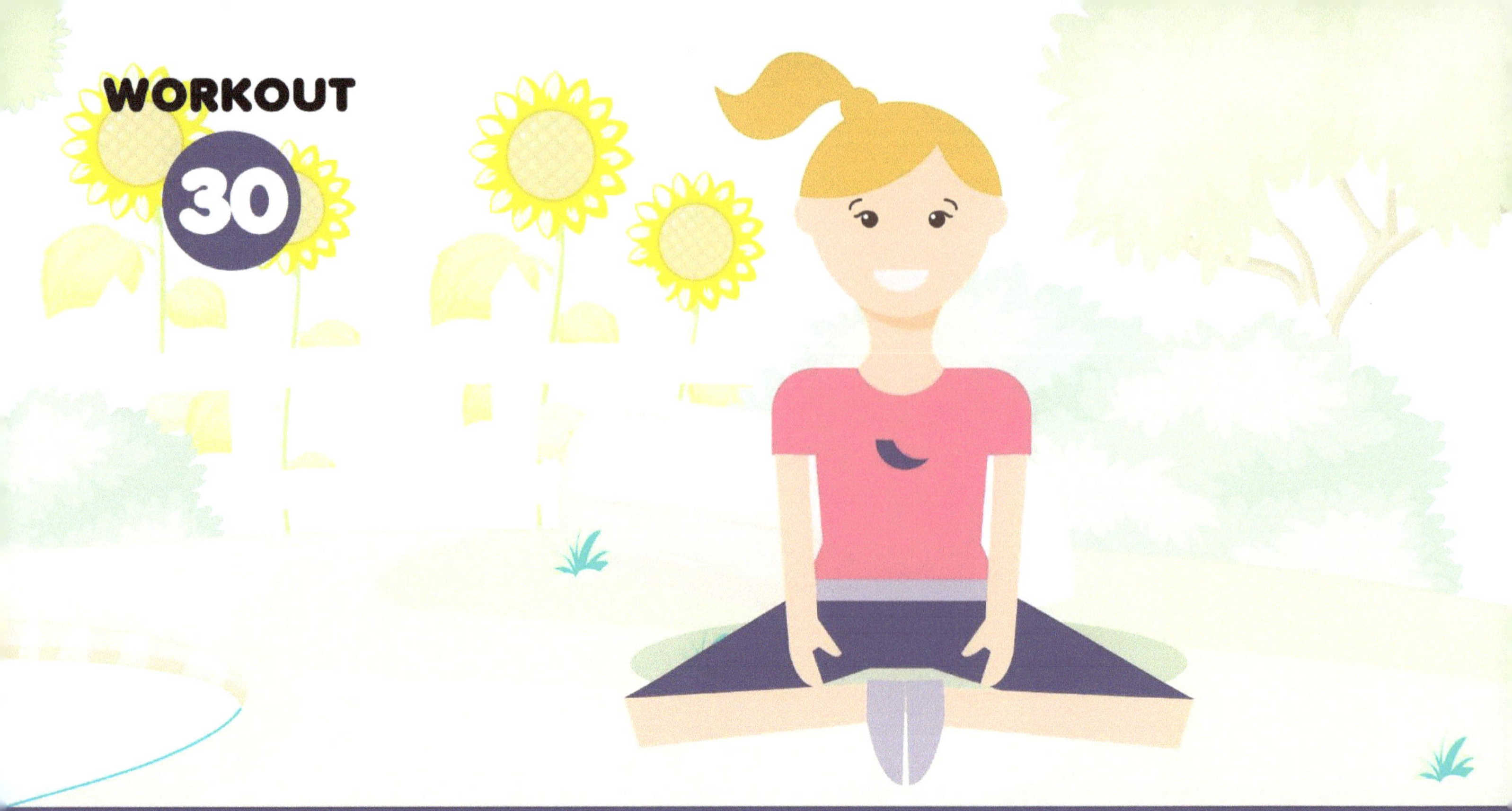

BUTTERFLY STRETCH

HOW LONG?

45

SECS

HOW TO DO IT

Sitting, bring the bottoms of your feet together. Pull feet as close to your hips as you can tolerate. Holding your feet, lean forward slightly. Hold.

The stretch that makes your groin muscle cry with happiness.

READY FOR THE NEXT ONE?

WORKOUT

31

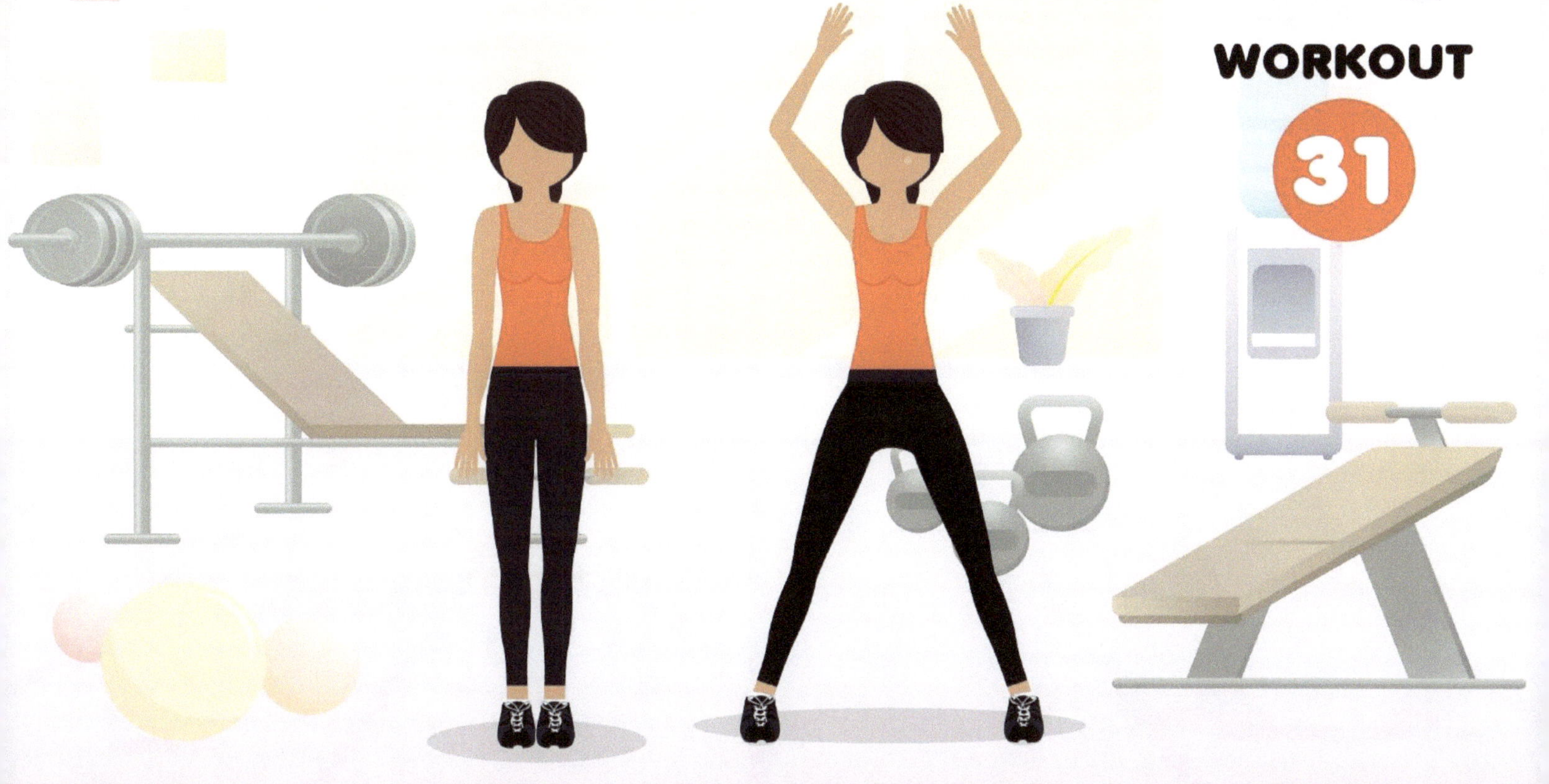

JUMPING JACKS

HOW MANY?

25

HOW TO DO IT

Stand, arms at side.
Jump, spreading your legs out and lift arms to the sky at same time. Modified version is stepping out, alternating legs.

The exercise women won't want to do without a bra.

READY FOR THE NEXT ONE? ➡

WORKOUT

32

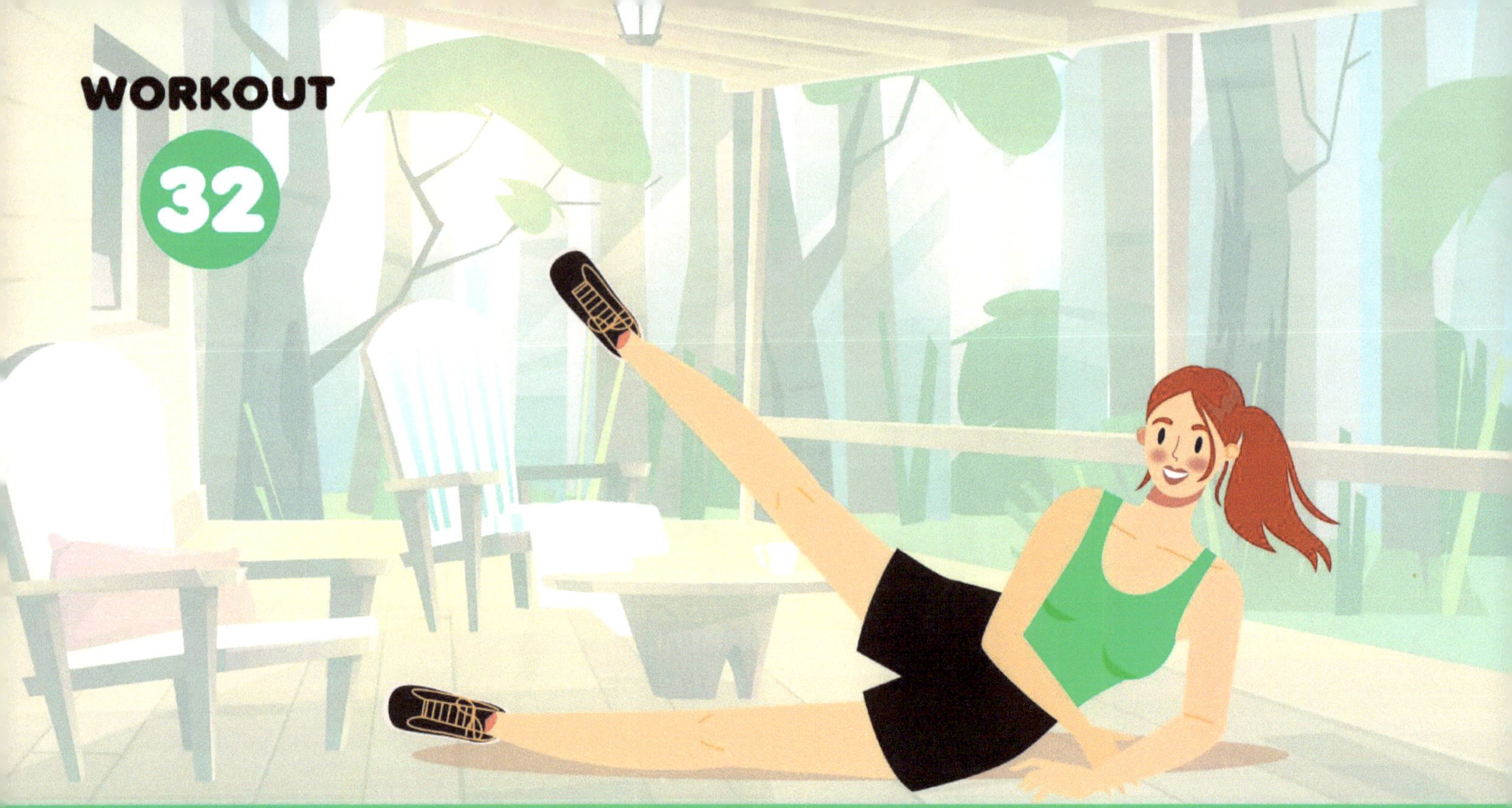

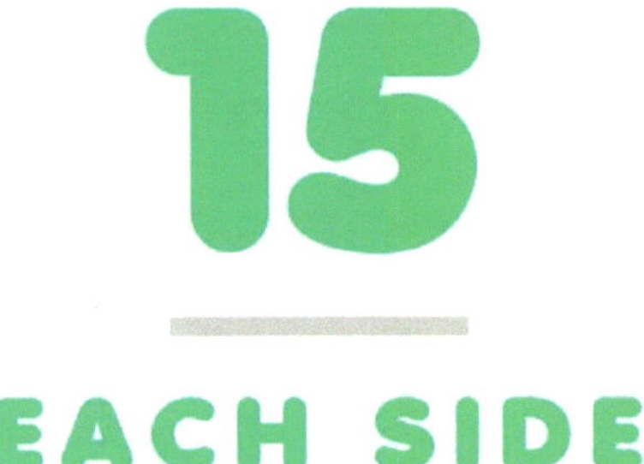

SIDE LEG LIFTS

HOW MANY?

15

EACH SIDE

HOW TO DO IT

Lie on your side, elbow bracing you up. Lift your leg in the air and back down.

Be prepared to have a hard time getting out of bed tomorrow morning.

READY FOR THE NEXT ONE? ➡

WORKOUT

33

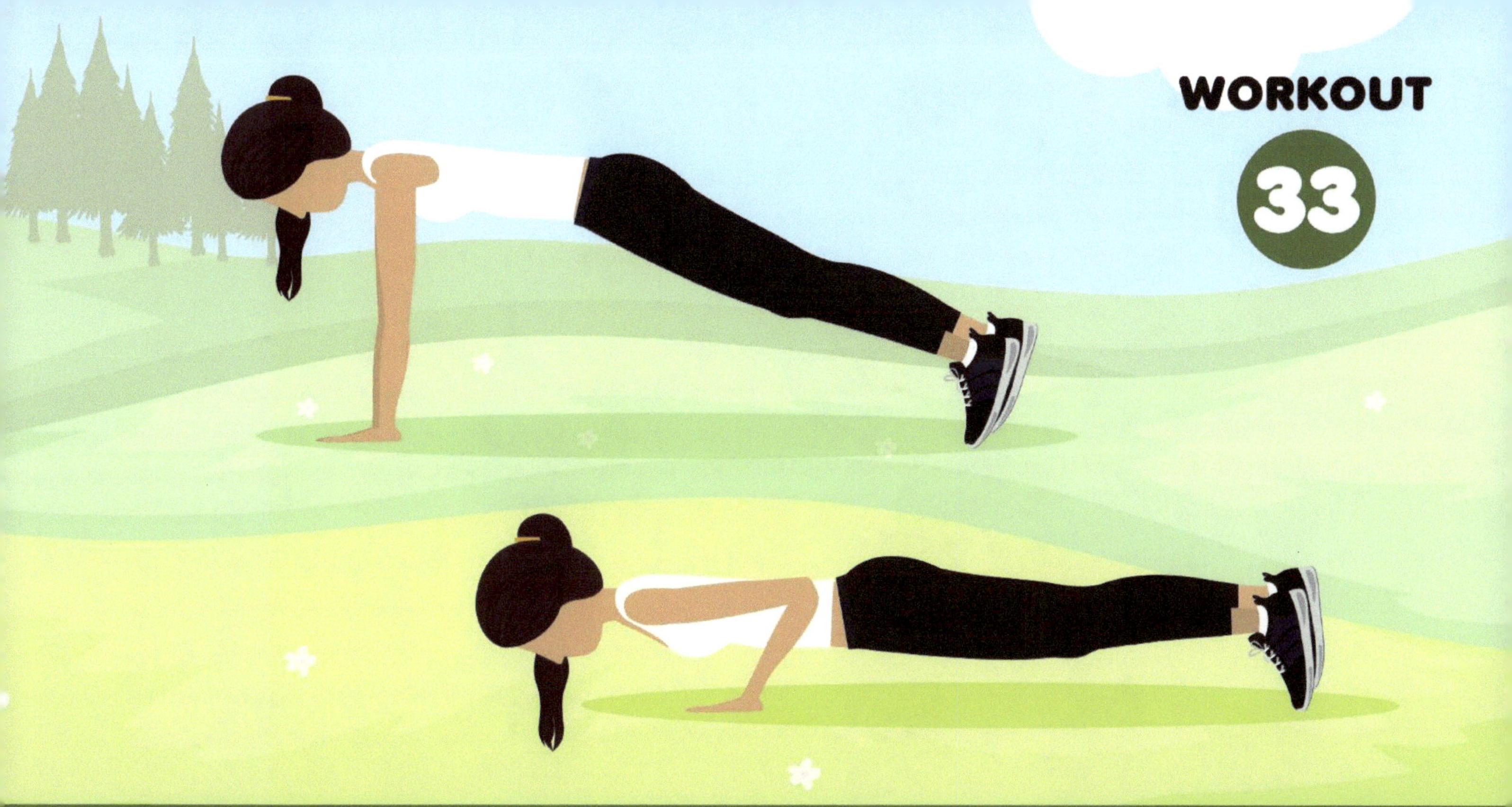

PUSHUPS

HOW MANY?

20

HOW TO DO IT

Get in plank position (on knees or feet), dip your elbows to go down and push back up again.

Future goal is to have your boobs hit the floor before your stomach does.

READY FOR THE NEXT ONE?

WORKOUT

34

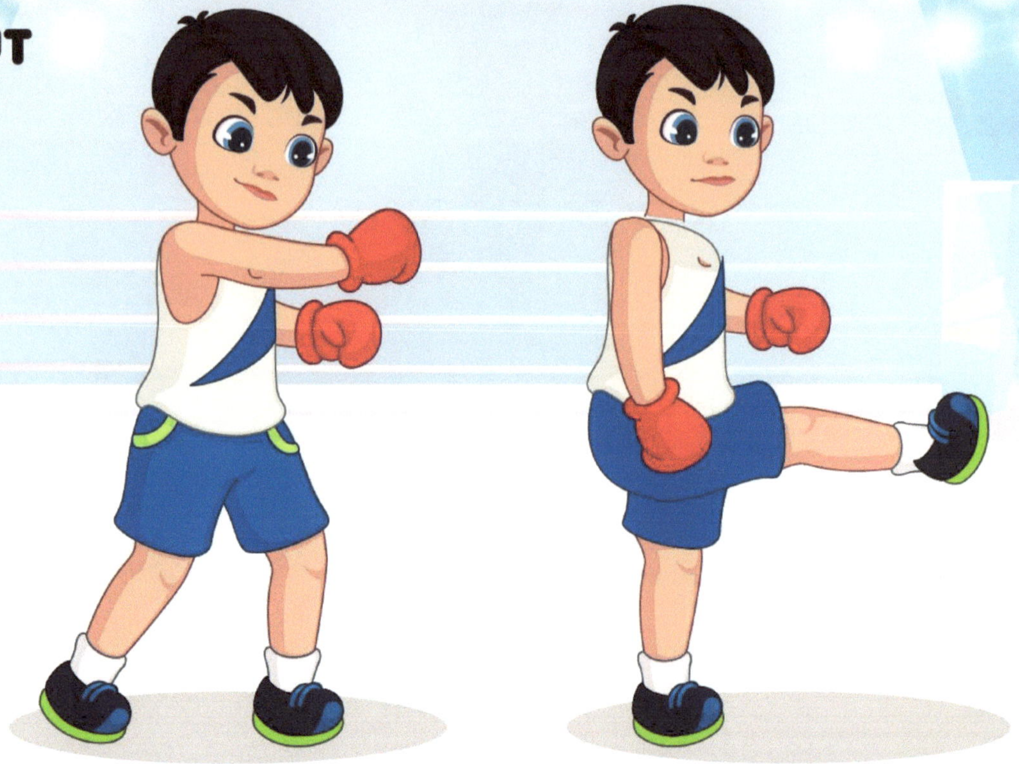

HOOK PUNCH WITH KICKS

HOW MANY?

10

HOW TO DO IT

Right hook punch, left hook punch. Right kick, left kick. (Counts as 1) Hook punch each arm, then front kick each leg.

A hook punch is like sliding your arm across a table while trying to knock someone's jaw.

READY FOR THE NEXT ONE? →

WORKOUT

35

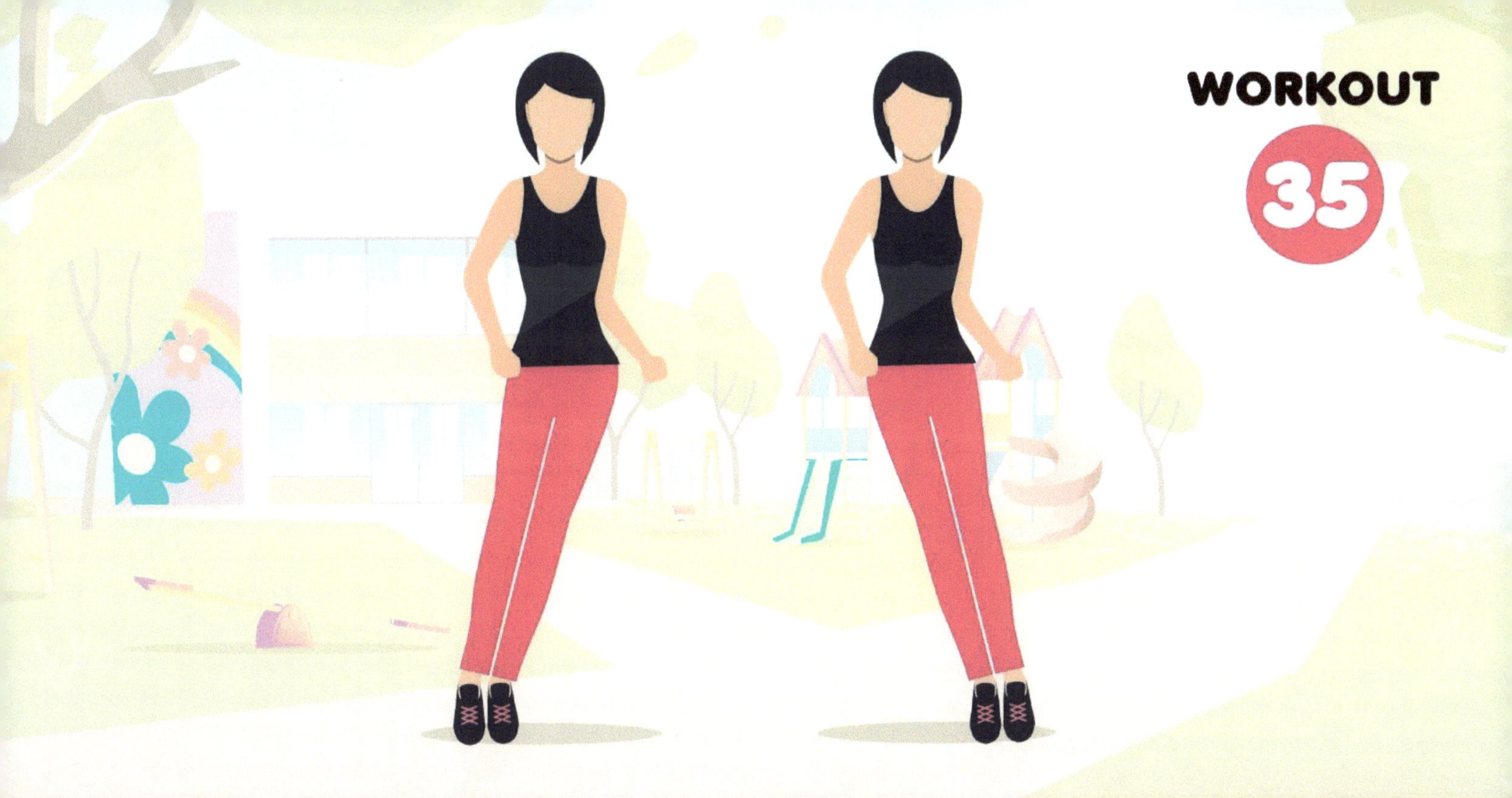

LATERAL HOPS

HOW LONG?

30

SECS

HOW TO DO IT

Jump side to side using your hips and legs only, upper body stays in one spot. Optional is to move forward and back in a zip-zag pattern, while jumping.

The difference between TRY and TRIUMPH is a little "UMPH".

READY FOR THE NEXT ONE?

WORKOUT

36

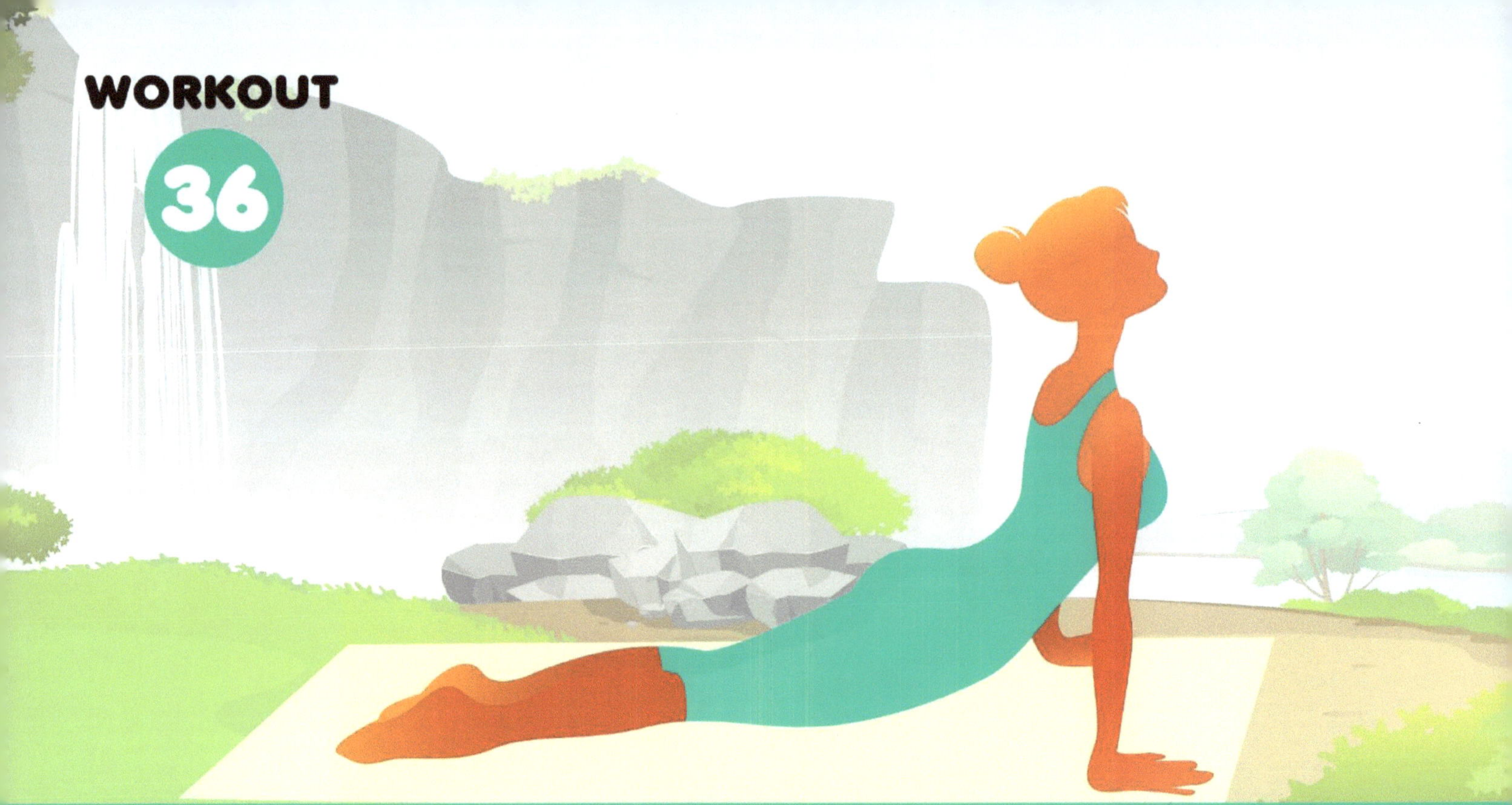

COBRA STRETCH

HOW LONG?

20

SECS

HOW TO DO IT

Start by lying on your stomach. Then bracing both hands on the floor, slowly lift your upper body. Don't lock your elbows. Stay in this position for the duration.

Better to bend then to break.

READY FOR THE NEXT ONE?

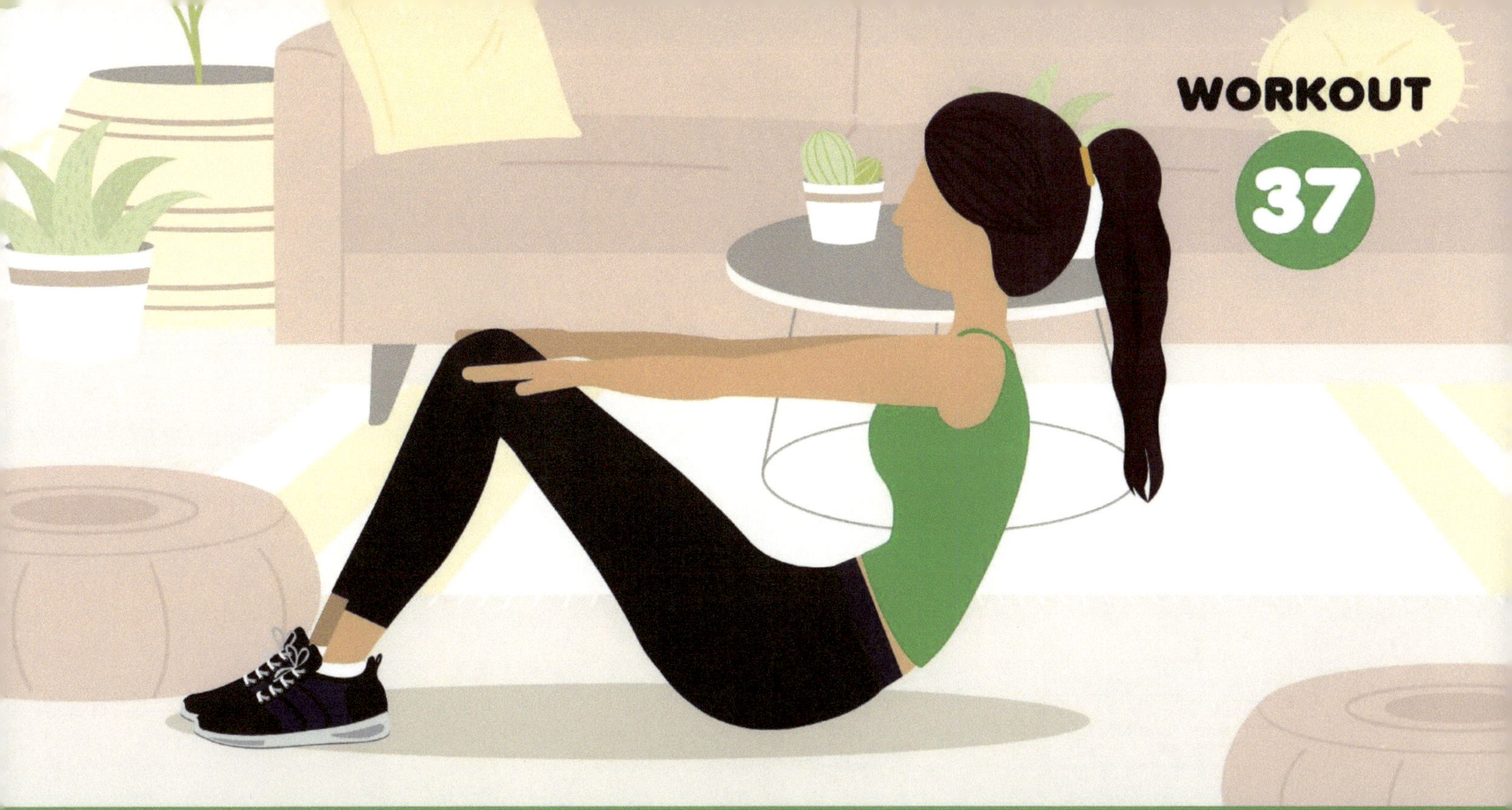

SITUPS

HOW MANY?

10

HOW TO DO IT

Lie flat on your back, feet flat on floor. Pulling yourself up with your abs to a sitting position. Lower yourself back down. Repeat.

It's time to stop covering our six packs with a layer of fat.

READY FOR THE NEXT ONE? 

WORKOUT

38

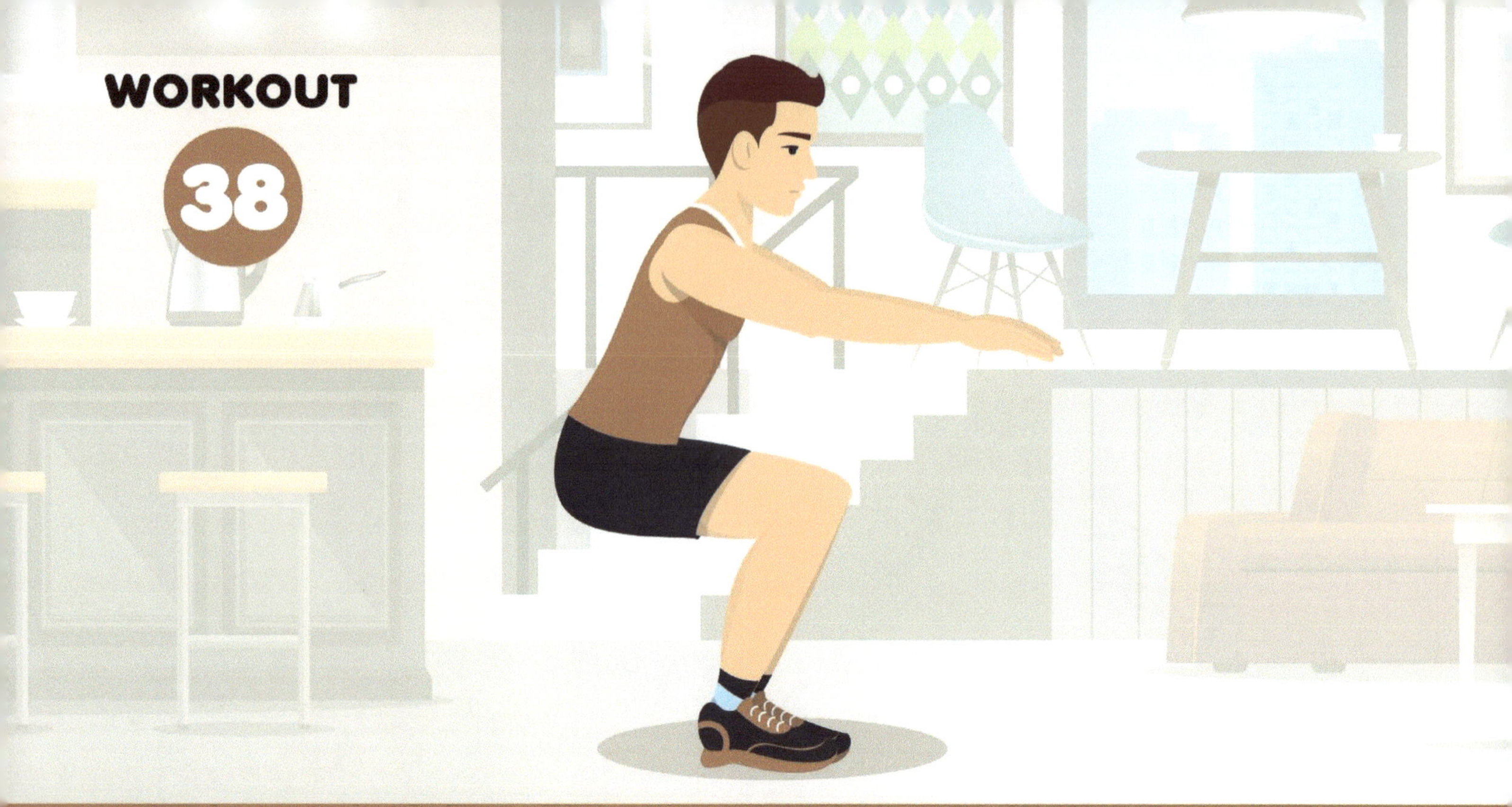

SQUATS

HOW MANY?

25

HOW TO DO IT

Standing, squat down like you're going to sit. Do not put the weight in your knees, stick your bum out as you drop down. Stand and repeat.

Squat until you walk funny.

READY FOR THE NEXT ONE?

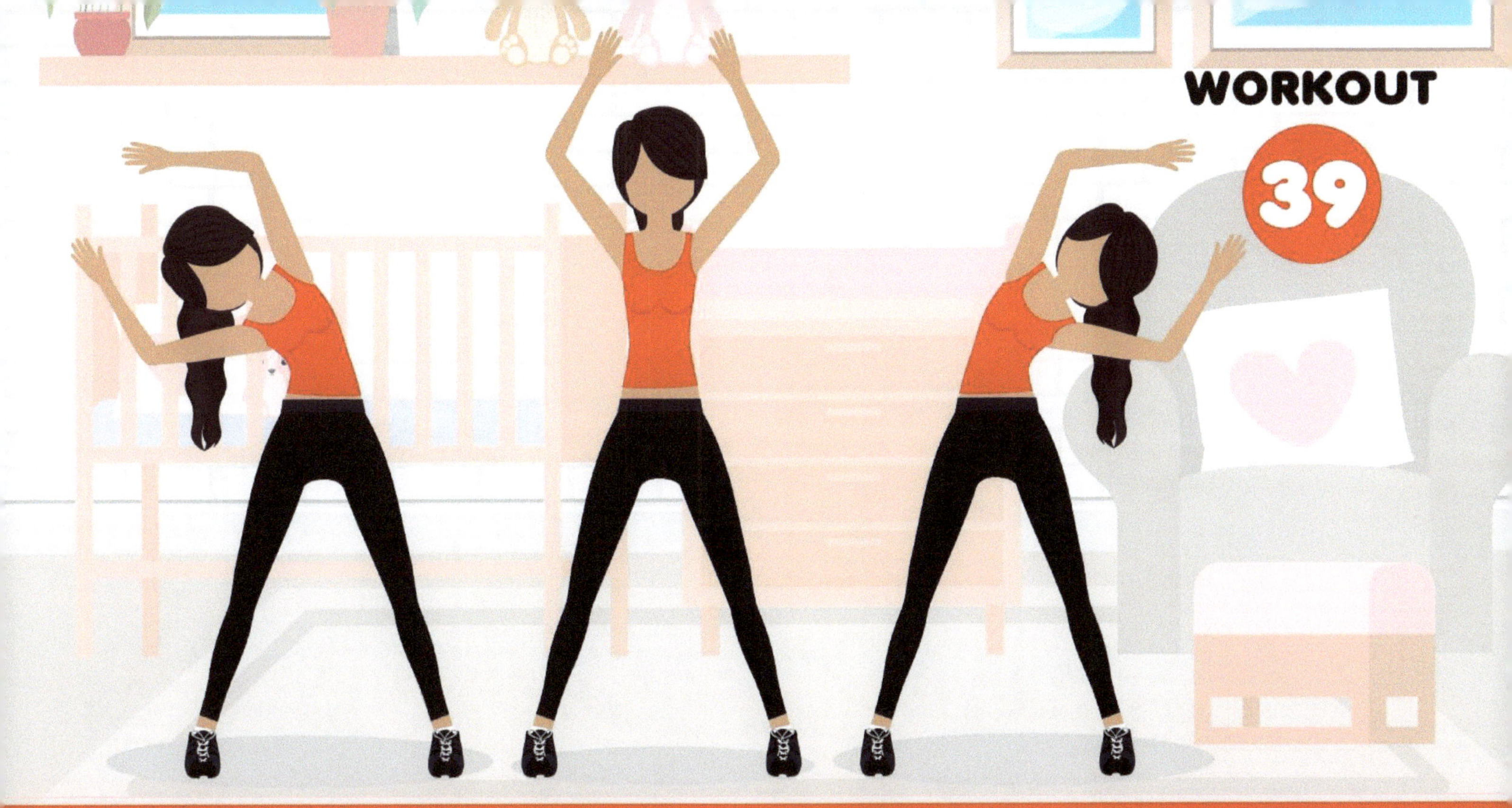

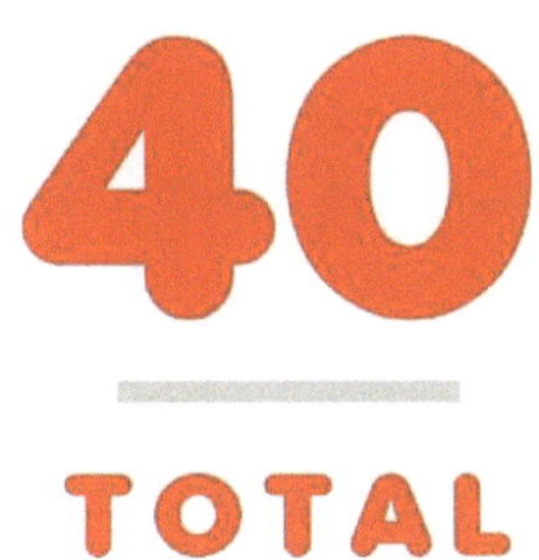

STANDING SIDE CRUNCHES

HOW LONG?

40

TOTAL

HOW TO DO IT

Standing, hold both hands up as though you are saying "stop!" Then bend to one side, then the other, alternating back and forth.

You'll feel like a rocking chair, but this exercise will help with those muffin sides!

READY FOR THE NEXT ONE? 

WORKOUT 40

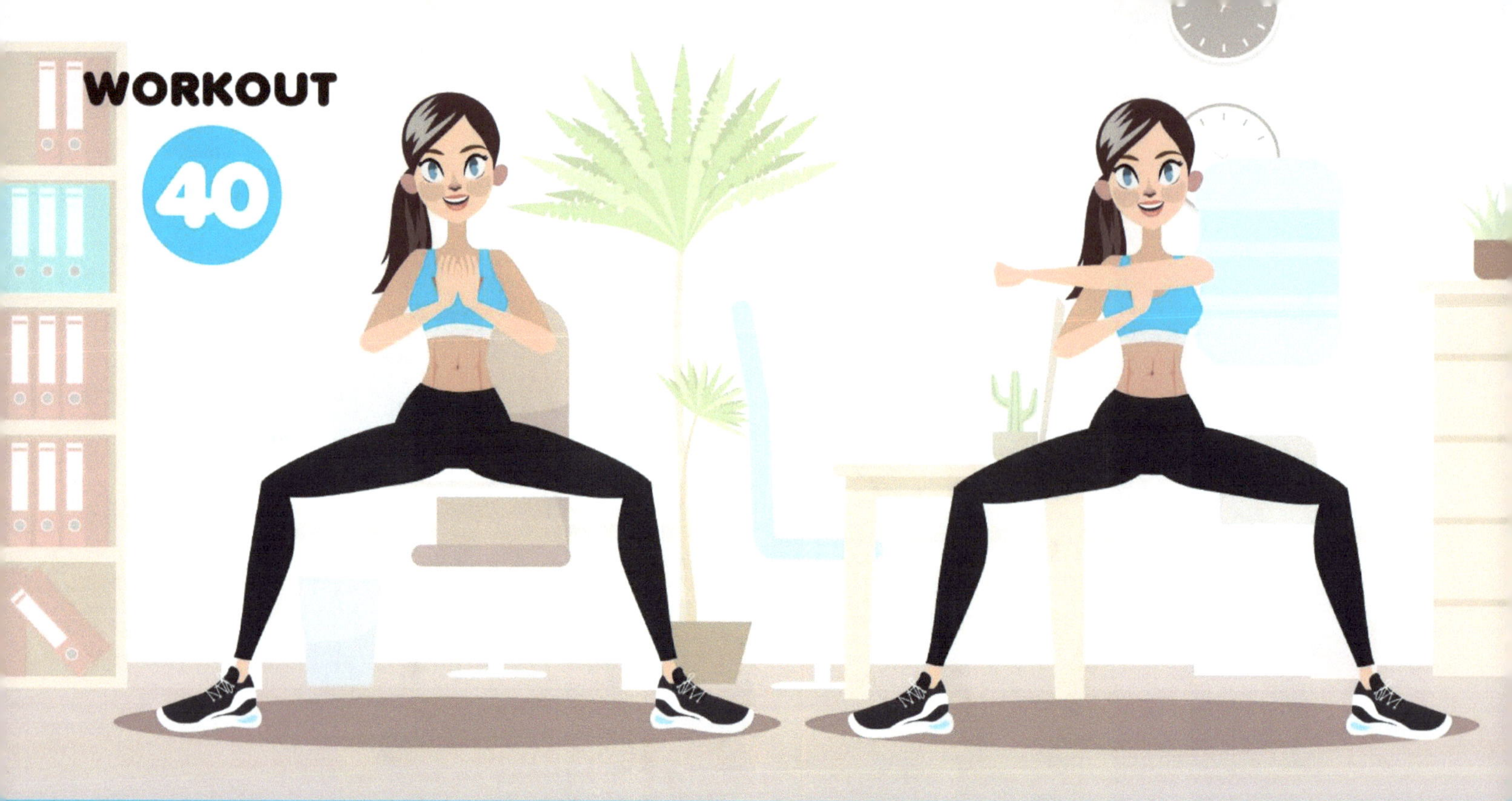

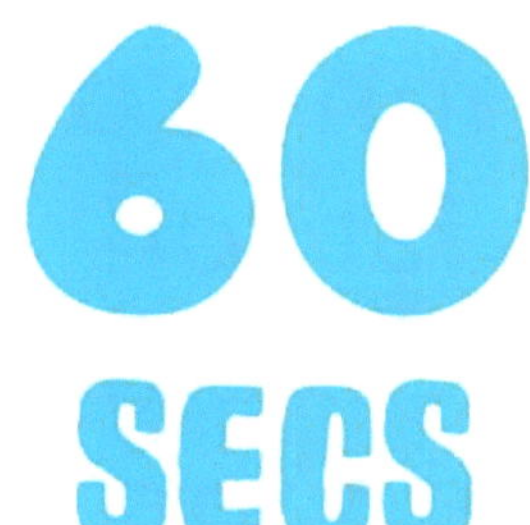

SUMO SQUAT PUNCHES

HOW LONG?

60 SECS

HOW TO DO IT

Squat down with your feet pointing outwards. Staying in sumo squat, alternate arms in a jab punch.

If you still look cute at the end of this workout, you didn't punch hard enough.

READY FOR THE NEXT ONE? ➡

WORKOUT

41

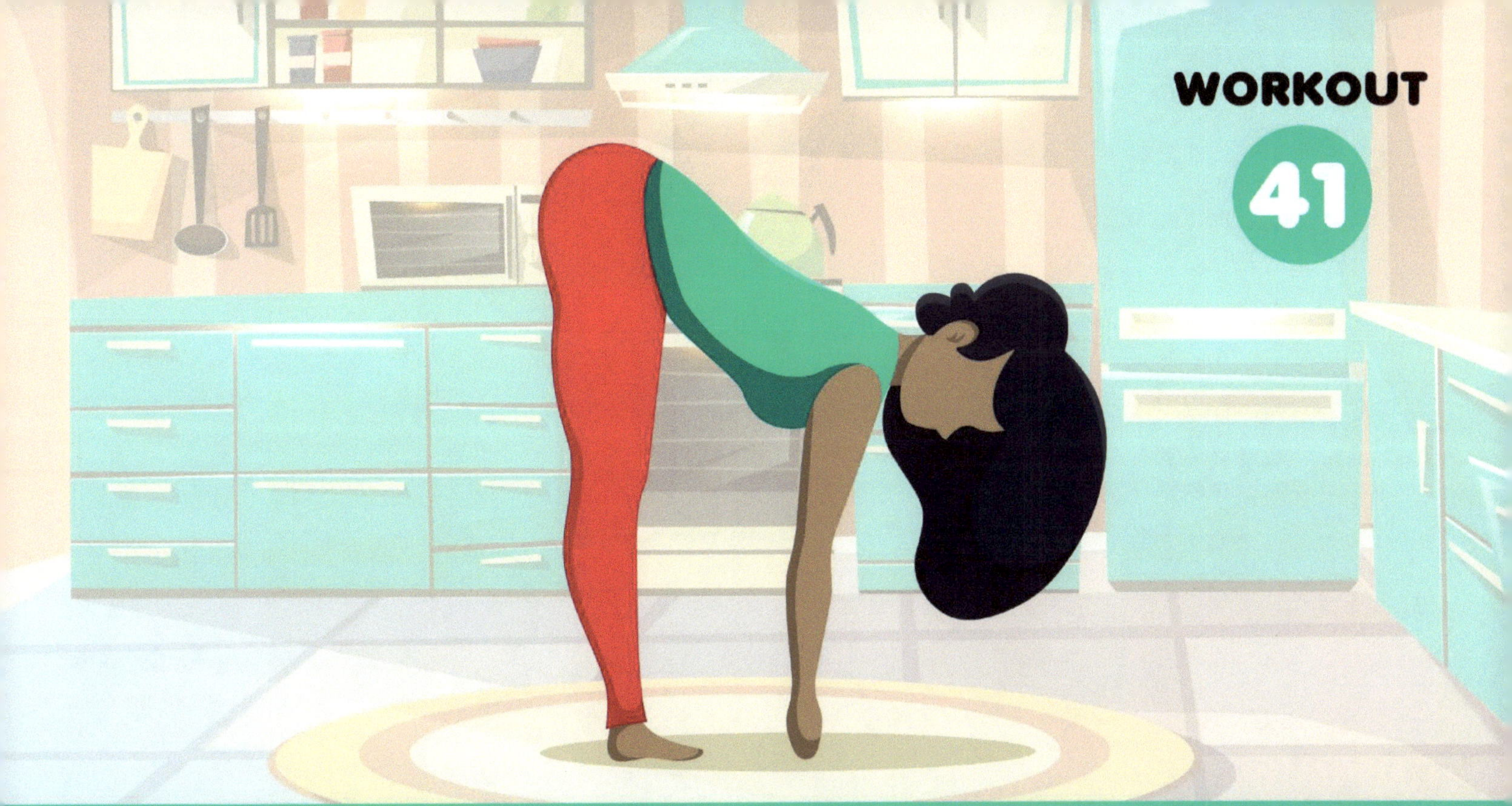

FLOOR TOUCHES

HOW MANY?

10

HOW TO DO IT

Slowly lower your body, sticking your bum out, don't lock knees when touching the floor. Hold for three seconds, then slowly come back up.

Relax into the exercise. Which means, don't use this moment to inspect the dirty floor.

READY FOR THE NEXT ONE? ➡

WORKOUT

42

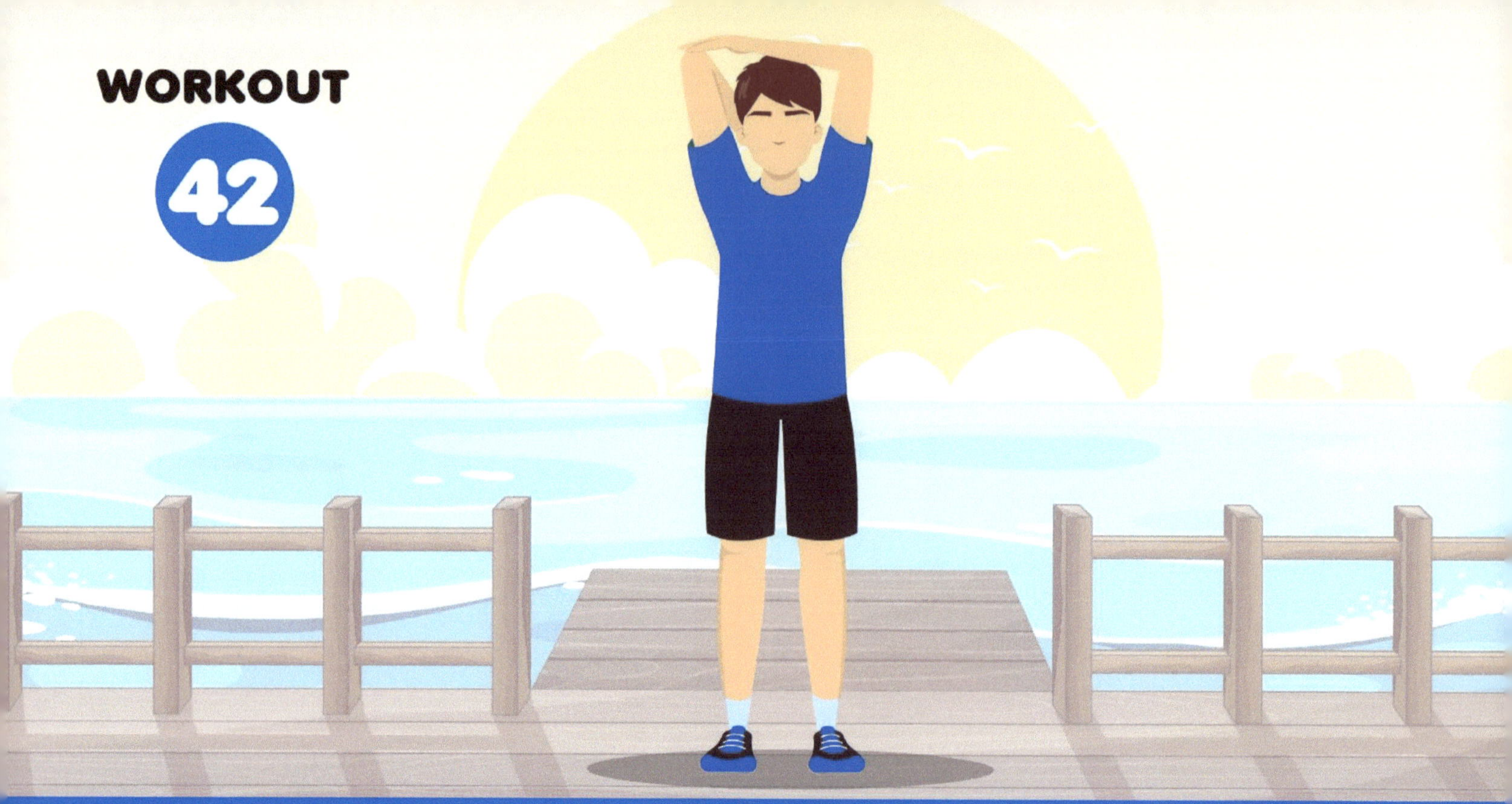

TRICEP STRETCH

HOW LONG?

20 SECS

EACH SIDE

HOW TO DO IT

Reaching one arm to the sky, drop your hand down to middle of back, keeping your elbow pointed up. Bring your other arm up to hold the elbow.

Take care of the triceps. You'll need to show them off in sleeveless shirts some day.

READY FOR THE NEXT ONE?

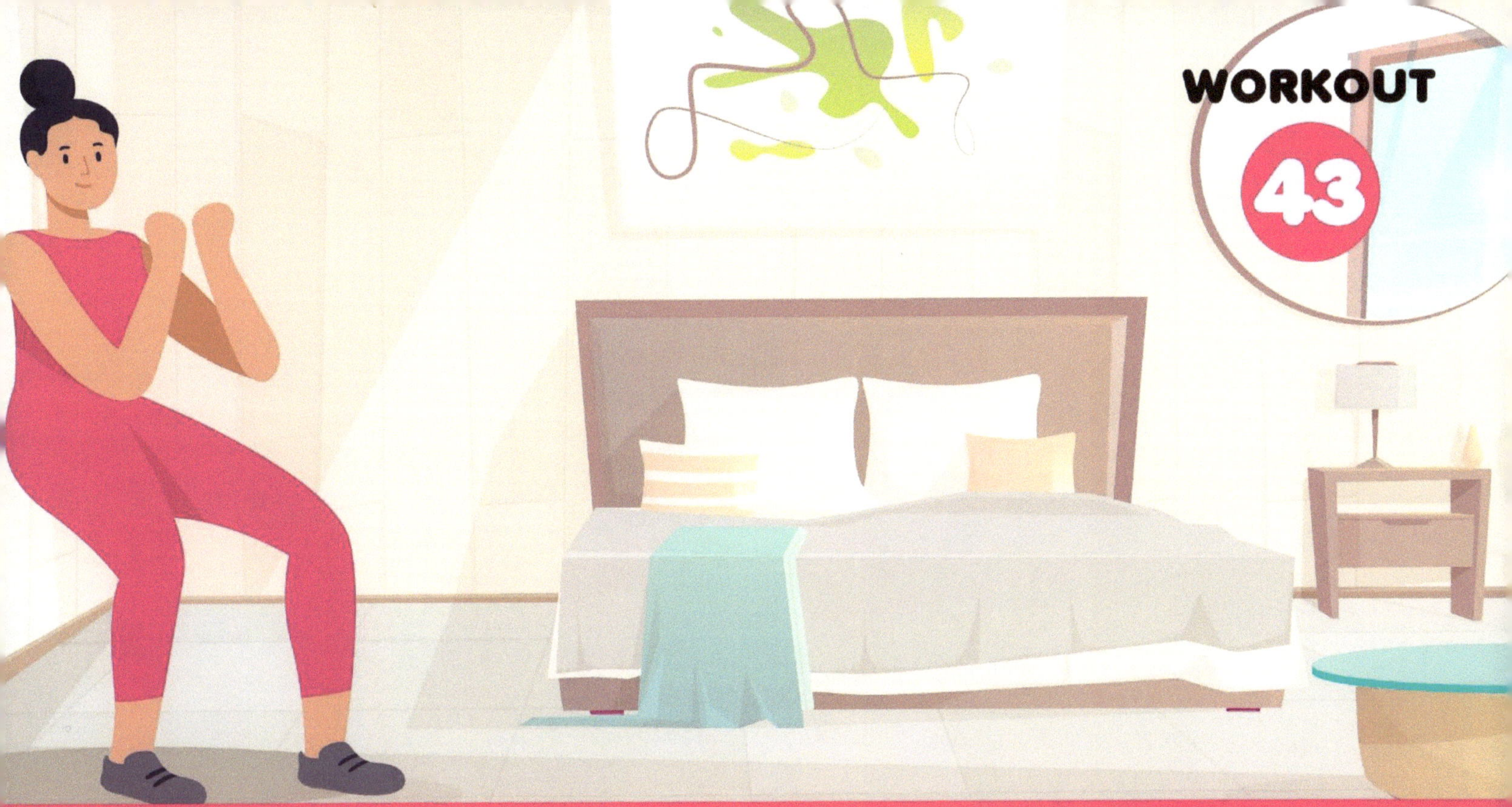

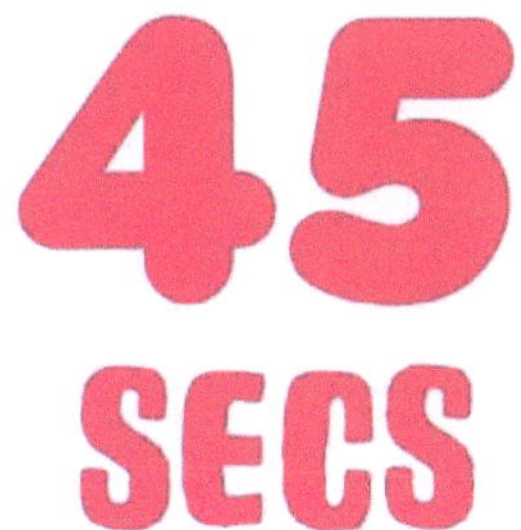

WALL SIT

HOW LONG?

45
SECS

HOW TO DO IT

Lean against the wall and sink into a sitting position. Hold.

If your legs feel like Jello, you did it right.

READY FOR THE NEXT ONE? 

WORKOUT

44

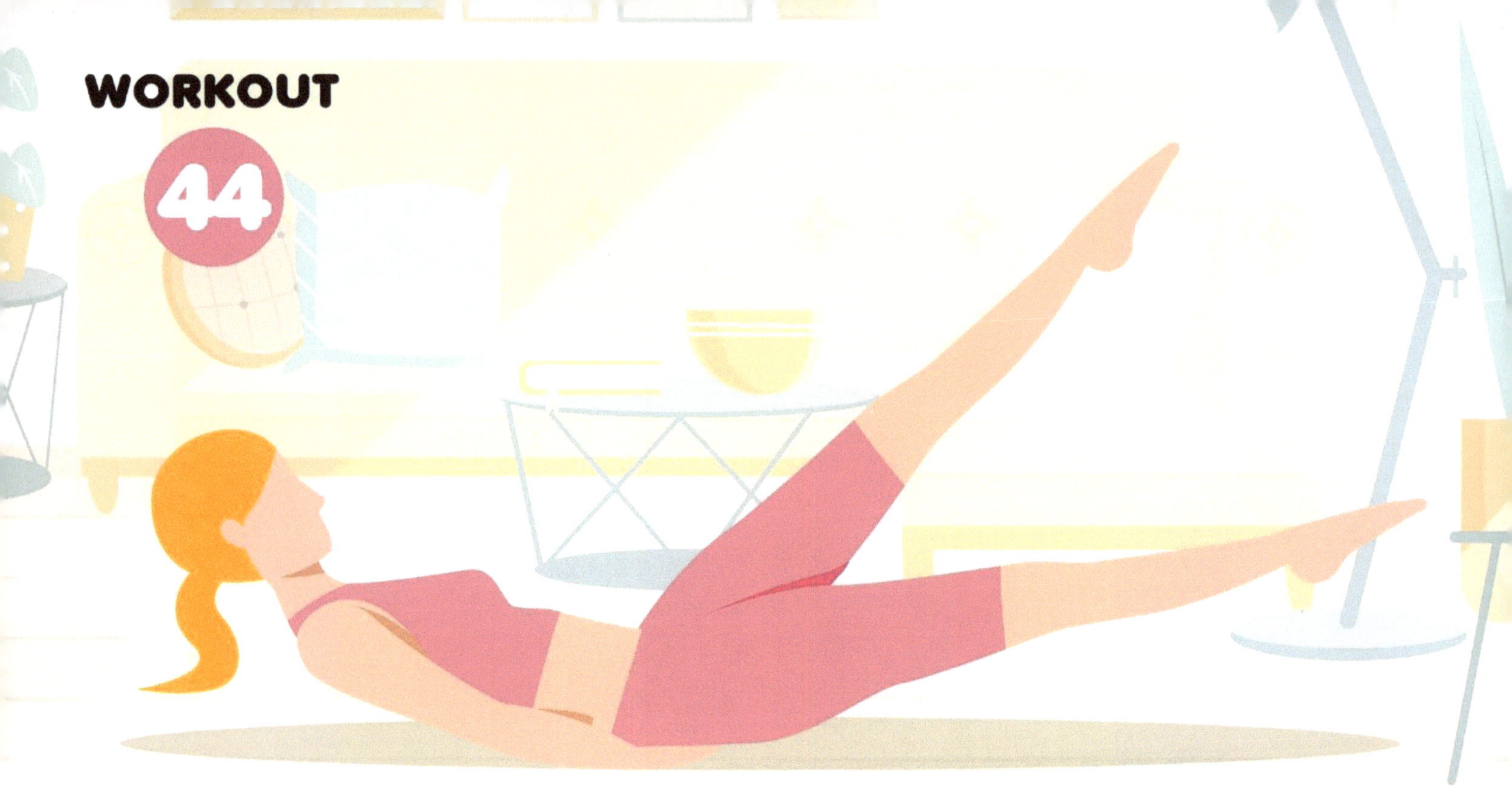

SCISSOR LEGS

HOW LONG?

30

SECS

HOW TO DO IT

Starting on your back, lift both legs in the air and then start “scissoring them” up and down. No legs should touch the ground until you’re done.

The only bad workout
is the one that didn’t happen.

READY FOR THE NEXT ONE? ➡

WORKOUT

45

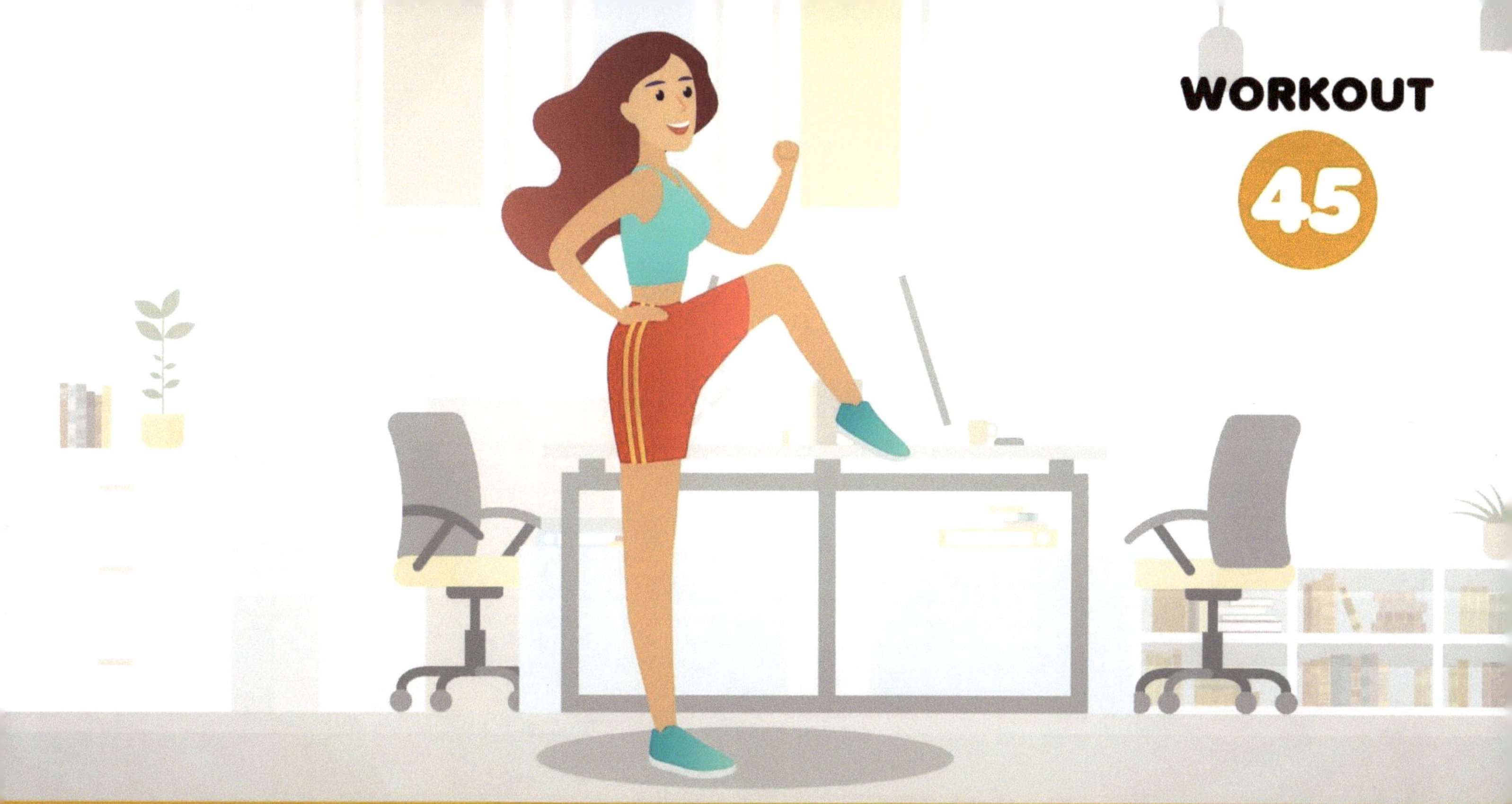

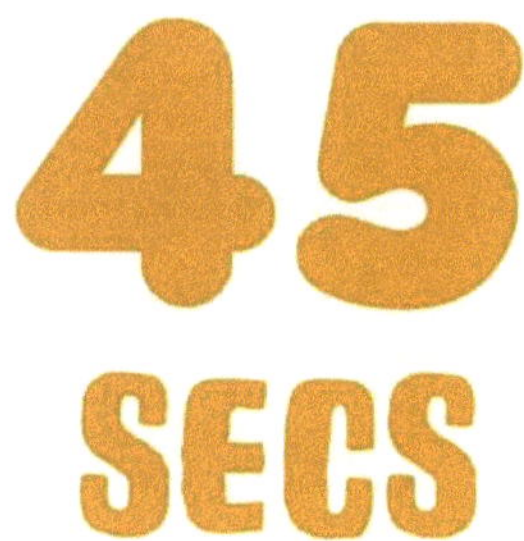

HIGH KNEES MARCH

HOW LONG?

45 SECS

HOW TO DO IT

March in one spot and swing bent arms. Make sure your knees go above your waistline.

Pump those high knees like you're trying out for a marching band.

READY FOR THE NEXT ONE? →

WORKOUT

46

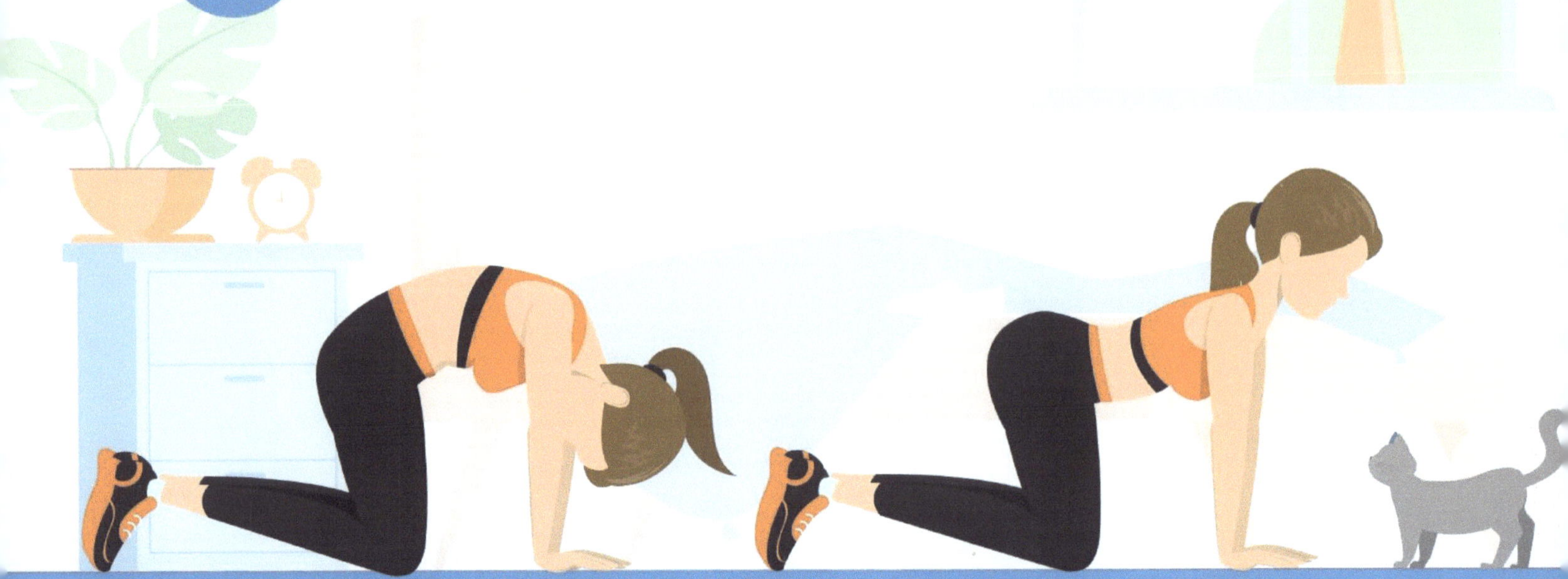

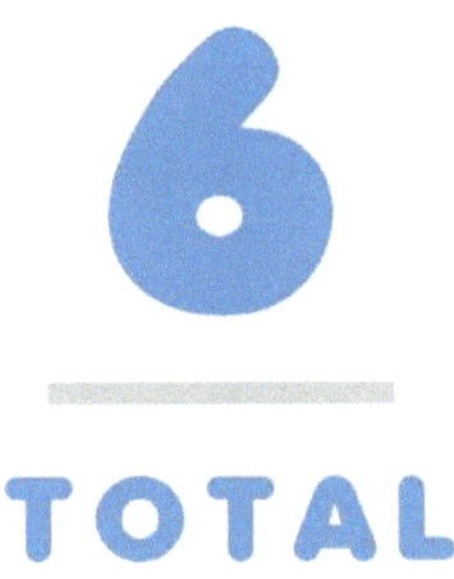

CAT-COW STRETCH

HOW MANY?

6

TOTAL

HOW TO DO IT

Get on your hands and knees. Cat - Round your spine towards ceiling and tuck your chin. Hold for 5 seconds. Cow - Arch your back and relax your belly. Hold for 5 seconds. Repeat.

A wonderful way to warm up your spine and look great doing it.

READY FOR THE NEXT ONE?

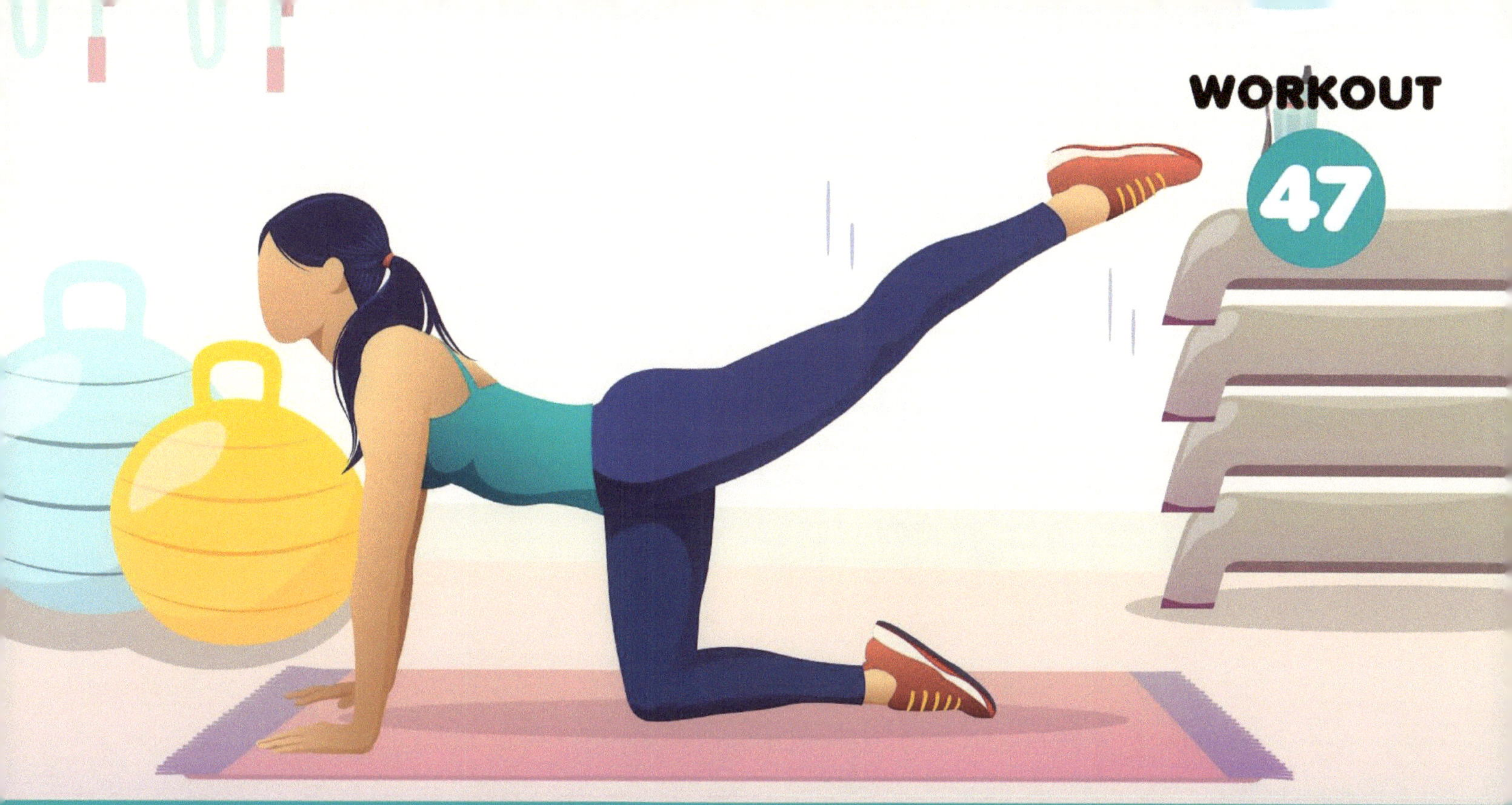

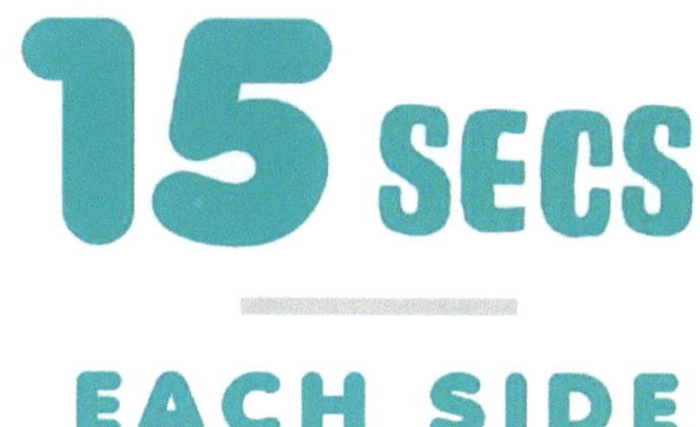

LEG LIFT PULSE

HOW LONG?

15 SECS

EACH SIDE

HOW TO DO IT

Get on your hands and knees. Lift one leg straight behind you, then moving it a few inches up and down, pulse it.

After leg workouts,
stairs just aren't the same.

READY FOR THE NEXT ONE? 

WORKOUT

48

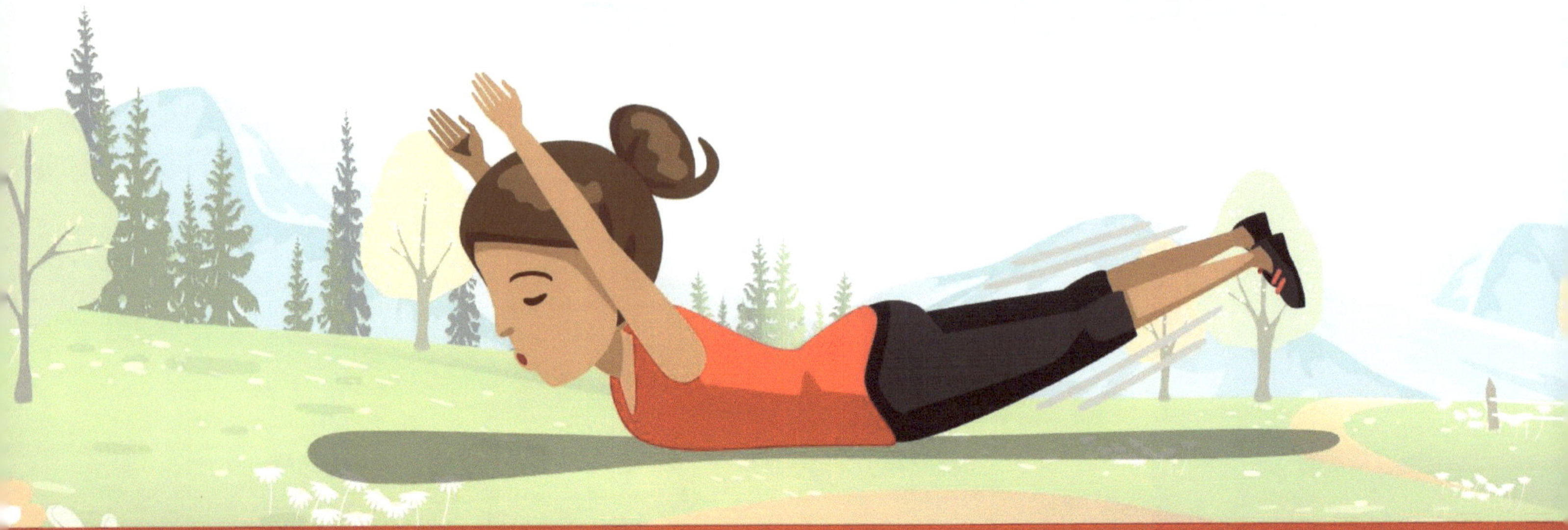

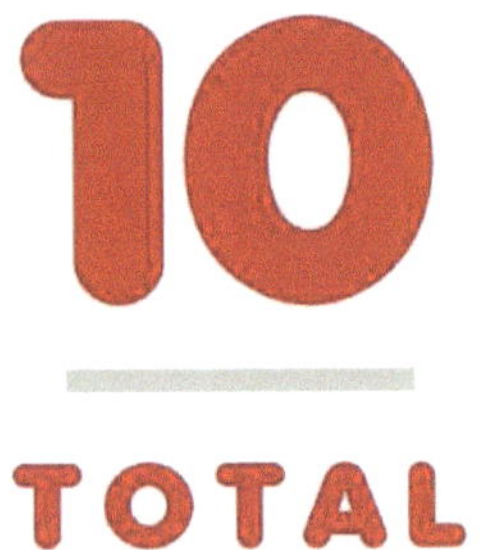

SUPERMAN

HOW MANY?

10

TOTAL

HOW TO DO IT

Lying flat on your stomach, arms extended, slowly lift arms and legs as high as you can. Keep your head facing the floor. Hold for two seconds. Come back down. Repeat.

Now you'll understand why Superman's back was so strong.

READY FOR THE NEXT ONE?

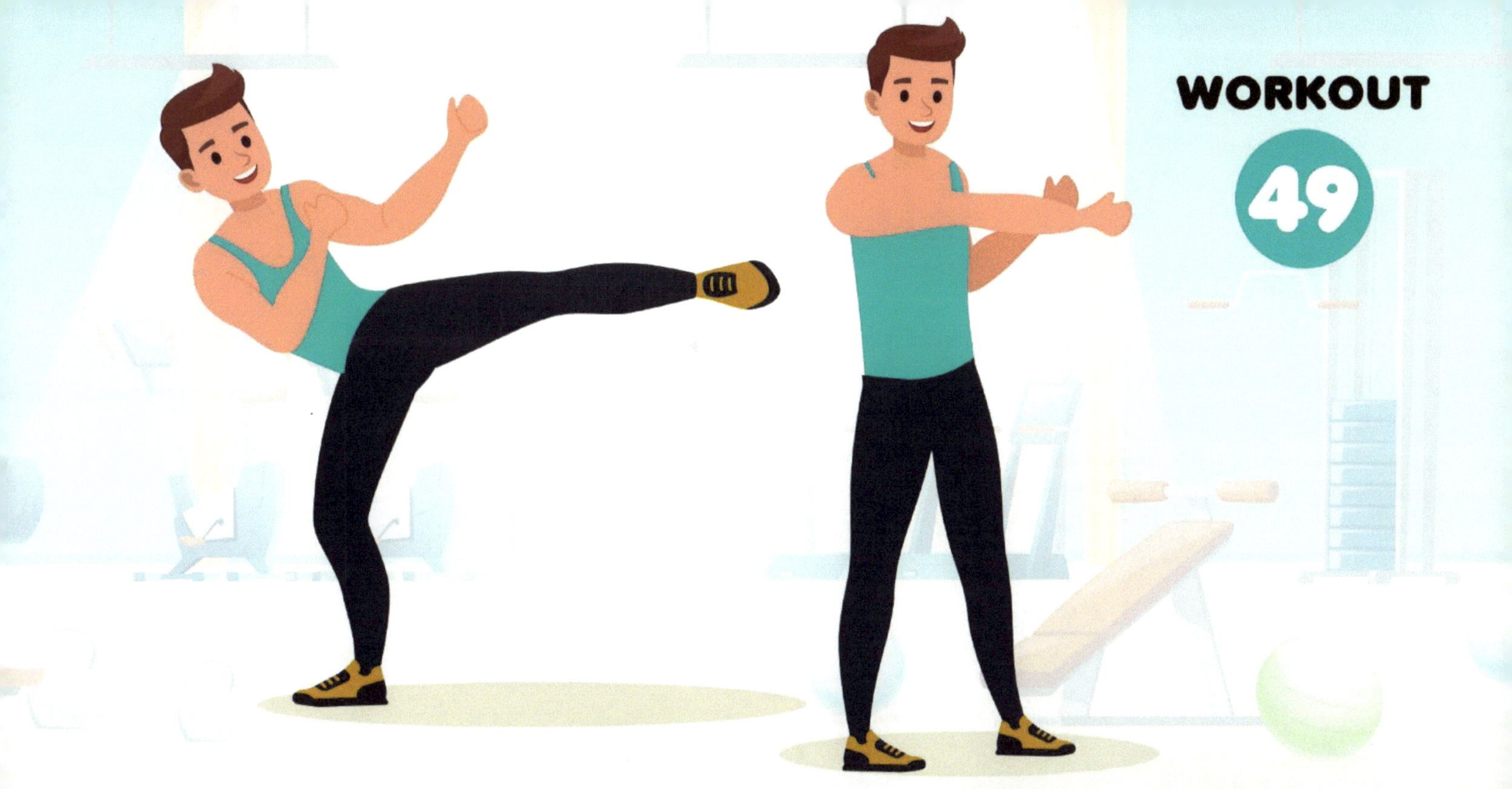

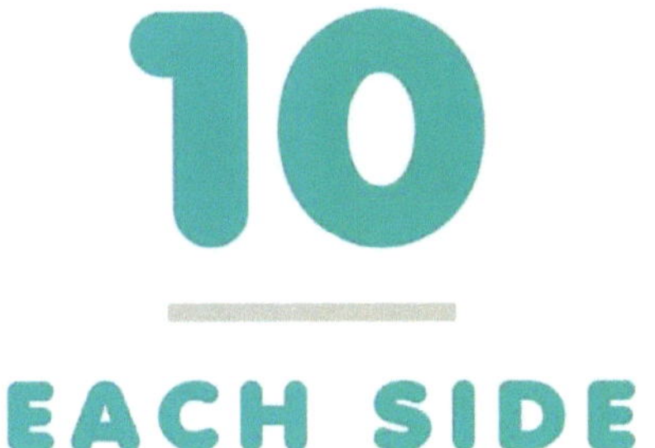

SIDE KICK WITH PUNCH

HOW MANY?

10

EACH SIDE

HOW TO DO IT

Side kick to the right, left arm should cross punch in same direction as kick. Finish one set, before moving to the other side.

Train insane or remain the same.

READY FOR THE NEXT ONE? 

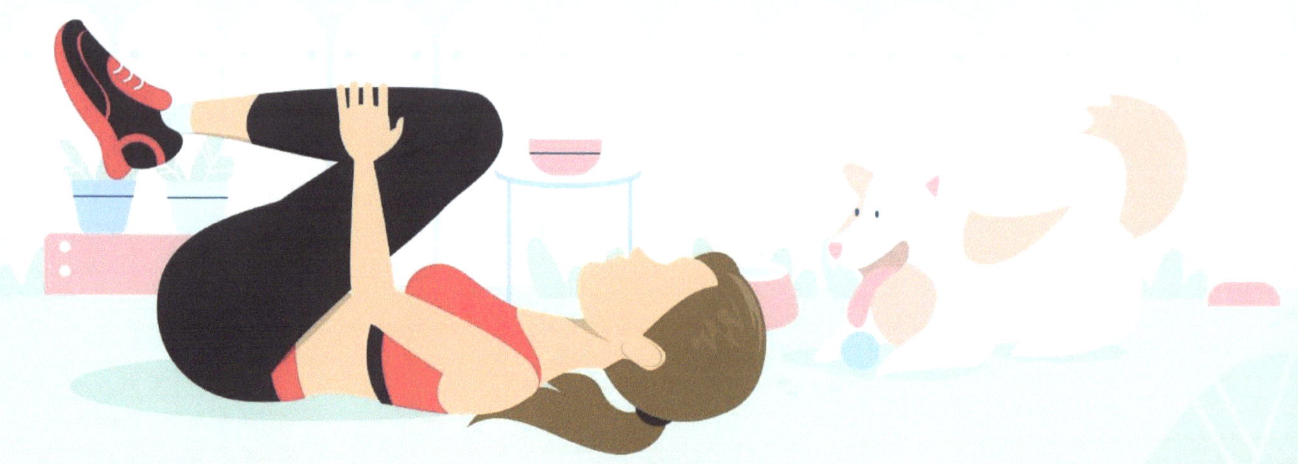

LOWER BACK STRETCH

HOW LONG?

30 SECS

HOW TO DO IT

Lay on your back and bring your knees up to your chest. Very gently rock side to side or stay in position.

Taking care of your back will have you bending like you're still in your teens.

READY FOR THE NEXT ONE? 

GREAT JOB, YOU'RE DONE!

Thanks for using my book

Squeezing in WORKOUTS

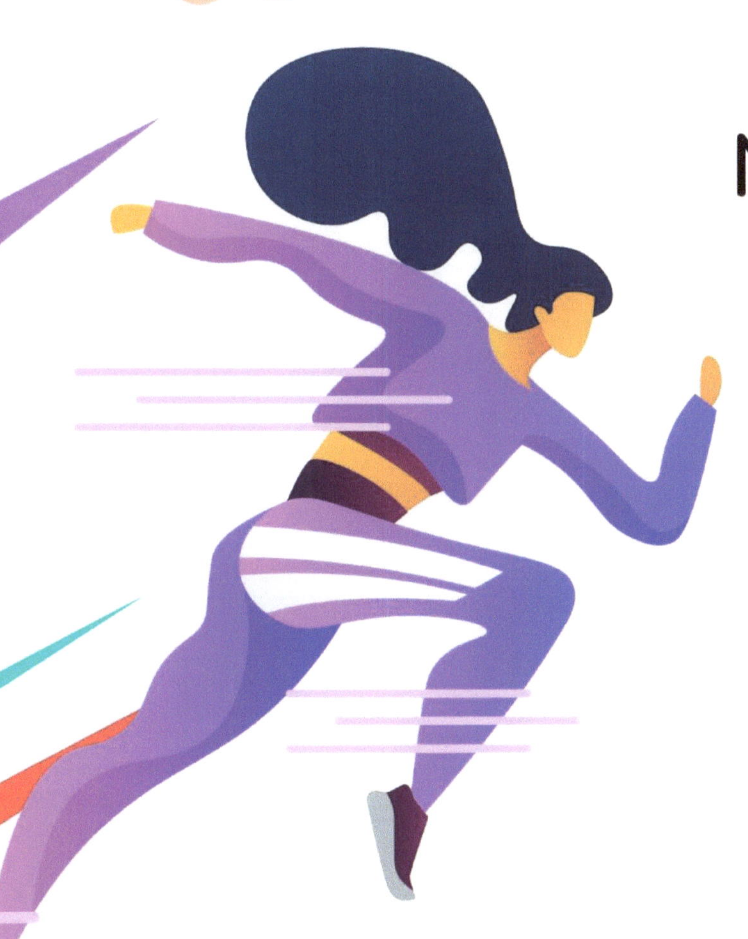

No matter how slow you go, you're still lapping everyone on the couch.

SO LET'S GO DO IT AGAIN!